Praise for *Evidence-Info*

M000279371

"Evidence-Informed Health Policy *is a significa_____ be written. The authors effectively integrate the policy process with evidence-based models and approaches. Each of the elements incorporated in this book is critical to understanding how policy evolves and why evidence is so important. While the policy process can be very messy, this book will greatly assist nurses and other healthcare providers in framing policy issues, formulating policy, influencing policymakers, and evaluating impact. As someone who teaches health policy, this book is an excellent asset for students who study health policy and the faculty who teach them."*

–Jean Johnson, PhD, RN, FAAN
Dean Emerita and Professor
School of Nursing
George Washington University

"Drs. Loversidge and Zurmehly masterfully combine the theoretical and practical aspects of policymaking using a tailored evidence-based framework that most nurses will find user-friendly and relatable. Examples of real-life policy issues are interspersed throughout, along with strategy tools and tables that further facilitate readers' under-standing of key policy principles. Evidence-Informed Health Policy *is an important book that educators and students can use as a foundational guide for exploring the role of nurses in policymaking and professional advocacy."*

–Janice K. Lanier, JD, RN
Nurse Educator/Consultant
Meredith Enterprises

"Evidence-Informed Health Policy *is a must-have resource for teaching and learning how to translate the language of evidenced-based practice into health policymaking. Drs. Loversidge & Zurmehly provide an innovative model for applying EBP to health policymaking and artfully guide the reader through a study of healthcare policy and politics. This will be the preeminent guidebook for nurses who work in health policy and is a must-read for those seeking to become health policy advocates."*

–Robin M. Rosselet, DNP, APRN-CNP, AOCN
Director of Advanced Practice Providers
The James Cancer Hospital & Solove Research Institute

EVIDENCE-INFORMED HEALTH POLICY

Using EBP to Transform Policy in Nursing and Healthcare

JACQUELINE M. LOVERSIDGE, PHD, RNC-AWHC
JOYCE ZURMEHLY, PHD, DNP, RN, NEA-BC, ANEF

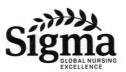

Sigma
GLOBAL NURSING
EXCELLENCE

The Sigma Theta Tau International Honor Society of Nursing (Sigma) is a nonprofit organization whose mission is advancing world health and celebrating nursing excellence in scholarship, leadership, and service. Founded in 1922, Sigma has more than 135,000 active members in over 90 countries and territories. Members include practicing nurses, instructors, researchers, policymakers, entrepreneurs, and others. Sigma's more than 530 chapters are located at more than 700 institutions of higher education throughout Armenia, Australia, Botswana, Brazil, Canada, Colombia, England, Ghana, Hong Kong, Ireland, Japan, Jordan, Kenya, Lebanon, Malawi, Mexico, the Netherlands, Nigeria, Pakistan, Philippines, Portugal, Puerto Rico, Singapore, South Africa, South Korea, Swaziland, Sweden, Taiwan, Tanzania, Thailand, the United States, and Wales. Learn more at www.sigmanursing.org.

Sigma Theta Tau International

550 West North Street

Indianapolis, IN, USA 46202

To order additional books, buy in bulk, or order for corporate use, contact Sigma Marketplace at 888.654.4968 (US and Canada) or +1.317.634.8171 (outside US and Canada).

To request a review copy for course adoption, email solutions@sigmamarketplace.org or call 888.654.4968 (US and Canada) or +1.317.634.8171 (outside US and Canada).

To request author information, or for speaker or other media requests, contact Sigma Marketing at 888.634.7575 (US and Canada) or +1.317.634.8171 (outside US and Canada).

ISBN: 9781948057202
EPUB ISBN: 9781948057219
PDF ISBN: 9781948057226
MOBI ISBN: 9781948057233

Library of Congress Cataloging-in-Publication data

Names: Loversidge, Jacqueline M., 1952- author. | Zurmehly, Joyce, 1957-
author. | Sigma Theta Tau International, issuing body.
Title: Evidence-informed health policy : using EBP to transform policy in
nursing and healthcare / Jacqueline M. Loversidge, Joyce Zurmehly.
Description: Indianapolis, IN : Sigma Theta Tau International, [2019] |
Includes bibliographical references and index.
Identifiers: LCCN 2019001827| ISBN 9781948057202 (pbk.) | ISBN 9781948057219
(epub ebook) | ISBN 9781948057226 (pdf ebook) | ISBN 9781948057233 (mobi
ebook)
Subjects: | MESH: Health Policy | Policy Making | Evidence-Based Practice
Classification: LCC RA427 | NLM WA 525 | DDC 362.1--dc23 LC record available at https://lccn.loc.
gov/2019001827

First Printing, 2019

Publisher: Dustin Sullivan
Acquisitions Editor: Emily Hatch
Publications Specialist: Todd Lothery
Cover Designer: TNT Design
Interior Design/Page Layout: Rebecca Batchelor

Managing Editor: Carla Hall
Development and Project Editor: Kate Shoup
Copy Editor: Todd Lothery
Proofreader: Gill Editorial Services
Indexer: Joy Dean Lee

Dedications

I dedicate this book to my loving family: my husband Bob, who is incredibly supportive and the most brilliant man I know, and my amazing daughter Katie. They keep me grounded. They are both my foundation and my inspiration, and the best things in my life.

–Jacqueline Loversidge

I dedicate this book to my loving husband Barry, who always supports and encourages me to follow my passions; you are the best thing in my life. To my children Erin, Erica, and Adam, who have given me many reasons to feel loved and committed to pursuing my dreams. I also dedicate this book to Brooklyn, Dylan, and Ruby, my loving grandchildren, who keep me young at heart.

–Joyce Zurmehly

Acknowledgments

I wish to extend my deep and sincere thanks to our Dean, Bernadette Mazurek Melnyk, at The Ohio State University College of Nursing. Without Bern's enthusiastic support, I would not have adapted the Melnyk and Fineout-Overholt EBP model for use in health policymaking, and the opportunity to write this book would never have presented itself. So, thank you, Bern! I would also like to thank my coauthor, who is also my great friend and colleague, Dr. Joyce Zurmehly. Joyce is committed to quality in all that she does and is unrelenting in her pursuit of any objective. We have learned so much about each other's gifts in this process that will make us even better partners in our future endeavors.

I must thank my husband, Bob, for his loving and endless support, for listening to me rant about the writing process late into the evening, and for bringing home many carry-out dinners, and our daughter Katie, who would occasionally force me out of the house for some respite. I would also like to thank Dr. Jeri Milstead, who offered me my first opportunity to publish on the subject of regulation and continues to do so. Dr. Ada Demb, who was my doctoral advisor and is now my good friend, has provided tremendous encouragement and also made me a much better writer with no thought for her own safety or mental well-being—thank you, Ada! To my good friends and colleagues Dr. Lizzie Fitzgerald and Dr. Edna Menke, I extend my thanks for your constant and unswerving support. I also wish to thank my cadre of awesome friends, Dr. Elaine Haynes, Eric Mays, and Rick Young; their wisdom and friendship have been invaluable in sustaining me through this process.

Another friend and colleague, who is gone but not forgotten, is the late Dr. Jill Steuer, who always encouraged my writing. I often hear her saying, "Give me another page, Jack." My heartfelt gratitude goes to Jan Lanier. Jan is a nurse attorney, and our association goes back decades to the time of the Ohio Coalition to Revise the Nurse Practice Act. Jan mentored me in the art and science of lobbying, but our partnership did not end there. Twice more, we found ourselves working together, most recently teaching health policy at the College of Nursing—me as a full-time academic and Jan as an adjunct, having retired from a life of service in a top-level position in a professional association. We remain "policy partners," and for that I am forever grateful. Finally, I would like to thank Rosa Lee Weinert, Executive Director of the Ohio Board of Nursing, retired, and a Past President of the National Council of State Boards of Nursing. Years ago, Rose took a chance by hiring an enthusiastic young master's program graduate into the Associate Executive Director role. She fueled my instinct that government regulatory agencies could do good work "for the people" and have a tremendously positive impact. She offered me both the guidance and the freedom to do that work.

–Jacqueline M. Loversidge

I discovered writing book chapters takes a lot of time, dedication, and perseverance, and the support of many. Of course, were it not for the continued encouragement and support from my husband and family, this may not have ever happened. My husband and children endured my many long days and nights of writing and listened to my never-ending stories about policy. With eyes glazed over, my husband pretended to listen and give feedback, but what I appreciated the most was his unconditional support and sometimes inquiring if I was going to be up late again. I am blessed with an exceptional supportive and loving family. In addition, there is one other person I know without whom this book would have never come to being: my co-author Dr. Jacqueline Loversidge. Jackie saw value in my contribution, which I would have never imagined possible. When I lost total faith in my abilities to make any type of a sensible contribution, Jackie was so kind and supportive with her phrase "awesome work." I would also like to thank Bernadette Mazurek Melnyk, Dean of The Ohio State University College of Nursing. She has such an encouraging and contagious spirit; she continually asks us, "If you could not fail, what would you do in the next five years?" This is my first of five years, and not only did I not fail, but I had a number of successes to celebrate. That was exciting to experience! A heartfelt thank you to all!

–Joyce Zurmehly

About the Authors

Jacqueline M. Loversidge, PhD, RNC-AWHC

Jacqueline M. Loversidge, PhD, RNC-AWHC, is an Associate Professor of Clinical Nursing at The Ohio State University College of Nursing. Loversidge earned a diploma from Muhlenberg Hospital School of Nursing in Plainfield, New Jersey; a BSN from Ohio University in Athens, Ohio; a master's degree with a major in nursing from Wright State University in Dayton, Ohio; and a PhD in higher education policy and leadership from The Ohio State University in Columbus, Ohio. She holds national certification as an ambulatory women's health care nurse through the National Certification Corporation.

Loversidge has been educating undergraduate and graduate students in the areas of health policy and regulation, evidence-based practice, and leadership in nursing and healthcare for more than 15 years. She has extensive experience in the regulatory setting, having held two positions at the Ohio Board of Nursing (OBN). The first was Associate Executive Director, which included the role of government liaison. Later, after a decade in practice and administrative settings, she served as the OBN Education Consultant, with the responsibility for oversight of all Ohio prelicensure nursing education programs. While at OBN, Loversidge served on various National Council of State Boards of Nursing committees, including the Committee on Special Projects, responsible for the transformation of the paper-and-pencil NCLEX licensure examination to a computer-adaptive model.

Loversidge has authored the chapter on regulation in Milstead's (now Milstead and Short's) *Health Policy and Politics: A Nurse's Guide* since its 3rd edition, as well as chapters on health policy and advocacy in Pearson's two-volume concept-based textbook. She is the author of the evidence-informed health policy model, which forms the basis of the model used in this book. Her scholarship interests focus on health policy, advances in health professions education and practice, and practice models that focus on improvements in quality and safety.

Joyce Zurmehly, PhD, DNP, RN, NEA-BC, ANEF

Joyce Zurmehly, PhD, DNP, RN, NEA-BC, ANEF, is an Associate Professor of Clinical Nursing at The Ohio State University College of Nursing. Zurmehly has been educating undergraduate and graduate students for more than 25 years. She is recognized for academic leadership in advancing nursing education through her work as a faculty scholar and nurse regulator. She has been influential in shaping undergraduate and graduate nursing education.

Zurmehly's primary area of contribution in nursing education has been in collaborating with state and national experts to set enduring nursing education policy by promulgating administrative rules. Because of her expertise in the regulation of nursing programs, she has been appointed to national committees, where she actively participates in developing policy in the regulation of nursing programs. She collaborated with the National Council of State Boards of Nursing (NCSBN) and broke new ground in nursing regulation by developing recommendations that promote collaboration with educators to foster innovations in nursing education. As part of this work, a model of the regulatory influences on nursing education was developed. Many have adopted these model education rules, thus positively affecting nursing education nationally and internationally. Zurmehly was also involved in the development of the Transition to Practice program at the NCSBN, in which multiple perspectives were addressed.

Table of Contents

Foreword

By Bernadette Mazurek Melnyk

Findings from a strong body of studies have shown that quality, safety, and patient outcomes can be substantially improved when healthcare is based on sound evidence from research. Yet, the translation of research into real-world clinical practice settings has been exceedingly slow, taking from multiple years to decades. Although many policymakers are starting to understand that they must base their decisions on the best evidence, the process of evidence-informed policymaking is also often painstakingly slow. Nurses, who are the largest healthcare workforce in the country, and other health professionals must understand the process of policymaking and how to best influence it with sound evidence from research.

This book by Drs. Loversidge and Zurmehly, two exceptional nurses and teachers who are seasoned in regulation, is a much needed and outstanding addition to the literature that fills a gap within health policy books because of the approach it takes with evidence as the essential foundation for policy. Masterfully organized, it starts with the origins of evidence-based practice so that readers can understand the basis and critical importance of evidence-informed policymaking. The content not only provides readers with the necessary knowledge of government structures, functions, and processes for the creation, passage, and dissemination of new bills but equips readers with the nuts and bolts of the seven-step evidence-based practice process applied to health policy, a pioneering first for the field.

This book should be a must-read in academic health professional programs and a staple in the library of every health professional. It is an exquisite masterpiece and a practical guide for how best to use evidence to influence health policy to ultimately improve the state of healthcare and population health outcomes across the nation.

–Bernadette Mazurek Melnyk, PhD, RN, APRN-CNP, FAANP, FNAP, FAAN
Vice President for Health Promotion
University Chief Wellness Officer
Dean and Professor, College of Nursing
Professor of Pediatrics and Psychiatry, College of Medicine
Executive Director, the Helene Fuld Health Trust National Institute for
Evidence-Based Practice in Nursing and Healthcare
The Ohio State University

Introduction

"Science and policy-making thrive on challenge and questioning;
they are vital to the health of inquiry and democracy."

–Nicholas Stern

The source of this quote, Professor Lord Nicholas Stern, the IG Patel Chair
of Economics and Government and Director of the India Observatory at the
London School of Economics, may not be well known by most nurses and
healthcare professionals. Nevertheless, the quote no doubt resonates with
those of us in healthcare who believe strongly in evidence-based practice (EBP)
as it applies to policymaking. Science and healthcare thrive on these same
principles, so it should not be a leap to appreciate the importance of challenge,
questioning, and science to health policymaking in a democracy.

Stern's observation is central to this book, which explores the world of
evidence-informed policymaking in nursing and healthcare. Nurses have long
been involved in healthcare as political activists. Indeed, our history is rich
with examples, from Florence Nightingale's work at Scutari and Clara Bar-
ton's during the Civil War, to the policy agendas advanced by contemporary
healthcare organizations. Nurses and other healthcare providers have spoken
out for positive change in policy, either as citizens and constituents or as members of their professional associations. Nurses, often in partnership with other
healthcare professionals, have influenced changes in reimbursement and scopes
of practice for advanced practice nurses, the provision of affordable healthcare
for underserved populations, improvements in workplace safety in healthcare
environments, and many other issues dictated by state or federal policy. For
years, nurses have shown up in force on The Hill in Washington, DC, and
at statehouses across the nation to make their voices heard. We have been
proponents for some pieces of legislation and opponents of others. Nurses and
other healthcare professionals also serve diligently behind the scenes as active
members of their associations and on their legislative and government relations
committees.

Whether we are inclined to be activists or more quietly involved—not everyone
is of activist fiber—every nurse and healthcare professional has a responsibility
to understand the current health policymaking environment. What happens
in health policy at the state or federal level affects the patients we care for, our
practice, and ourselves. On a personal level, our livelihoods are at stake, as

well as our own health; at one time or another, we will all be patients, as will those we love. When that happens, we all hope that the best possible policy is driving the care we or our loved ones receive!

As healthcare has advanced to drive responsible change in clinical practice by a body of scientific evidence, nurses and other health professionals are continuing to gain competency in EBP. This movement has aligned with a parallel progression in the science of policymaking. This is not an oxymoron. Health services research and health policy scholars have long argued for the use of scientific evidence to drive sensible policy. Over the last decade, the language in that discipline has evolved from the term *evidence-based,* which is used for good reasons in healthcare, to the term *evidence-informed* to acknowledge the realities of policymaking. When evidence is used in the world of politics, the best one can hope for is that it will inform the dialogue and leverage the outcome.

As nurses and healthcare professionals are so passionately engaged in policymaking, it is time to bring their expertise in EBP into their work in policy. Nurses understand EBP; it works in the world of clinical practice. The models are clear and straightforward. But they are designed for clinical decision-making, not policymaking. This book was born out of the need to translate the language nurses know and use when applying EBP to clinical decision-making into a language for health policymaking.

Many descriptions and models of evidence-informed health policymaking appear in the literature, but the intended audience is largely health services research scholars. Therefore, the language is not as accessible to nurses and other healthcare professionals as is the language of EBP. One of the authors of this book, Jacqueline Loversidge, who has taught health policy to master's-level nursing students for a number of years (and who, along with co-author Joyce Zurmehly, also teaches doctor of nursing practice health policy), used the EBP model described by Bernadette Mazurek Melnyk and Ellen Fineout-Overholt in her classes to help students understand how to incorporate evidence into policy. The EBP language and approach was not quite the right fit, however; it needed to be adapted from the clinical to the political. With Dean Melnyk's enthusiastic support, Loversidge adapted the model for health policy.

Loversidge's model, called the evidence-informed health policy (EIHP) model, was subsequently published in the *Journal of Nursing Regulation*. Its intended audience in that publication consisted of nursing regulators and nursing educators—in no small part because of Loversidge's background in nursing regulation and her current role in academics. Since then, both Loversidge and Zurmehly have successfully used the model in their health policy classes to help students understand how to integrate evidence into the health policymaking process. A portion of this book describes the adapted model.

The goals of this book are threefold:

- To persuade readers that evidence-based or evidence-informed policymaking is not, after all, an oxymoron, and that perspectives on the use of evidence in policy are changing. To our knowledge, this is the first health policy text in nursing and healthcare in which evidence-based policymaking is the primary focus.
- To ground readers in policy and policymaking to a sufficient extent that it serves as a foundation for using the rest of the book.
- To present the EIHP model for nursing and healthcare, adapted from the Melnyk and Fineout-Overholt EBP model. This model can be used by nurses and other healthcare professionals serving in active policymaking roles, teaching health policy, or simply interested in the process.

The primary focus of this book is on policymaking in government, but principles and strategies presented can apply well in organizational settings. Mention of these applications is made throughout.

Audiences who can best benefit from this book include the following:

- Nurse leaders
- Nurses who are members or staff of professional associations and organizations
- Healthcare regulatory agency members or staff
- Other healthcare professionals

These audiences can use this book to familiarize themselves with strategies for making the best use of evidence to leverage dialogue and influence policymakers to advance health policy agendas or as a tool to navigate governmental or organizational policymaking environments. It can also be used as a textbook for nurse educators and for nursing students enrolled in health policy courses. For educators and students, we anticipate this book will be particularly useful for guiding health policy-related DNP projects, which are an emerging interest and focus in DNP programs.

Chapters 1 and 2 of this book focus on the use of evidence in health policymaking and its evolution. They begin with foundations in evidence-based medicine and its extension beyond medicine to EBP. They then describe some of the most often used EBP models before segueing to an explanation of how evidence can be used in policymaking. Finally, they describe how the landscape in policymaking is changing to become more aware of and open to the use of evidence.

Chapters 3 through 5 provide a foundation in policy and government. These chapters focus on health policy basics and how policymaking works. They answer the question, what is health policy? They then describe government structures and functions that drive processes, followed by the processes themselves, using the US Congress and federal regulatory agencies as models. Theoretical models that are useful to understanding processes are also presented, including several that the authors find most useful in practice. These chapters end with a discussion of the influence of stakeholders and partisan politics on the policymaking process.

Chapters 6 through 9 describe the EIHP model. Chapter 6 provides an overview of the model as a whole. Chapter 7 describes its foundation, which consists of the first four steps: cultivating a spirit of inquiry; asking the policy question in the PICOT format; searching for and collecting the most relevant best evidence; and critically appraising that evidence. Chapter 8 addresses the next two steps: integrating the best evidence with issue expertise and stakeholder values and ethics, and contributing to the health policy development and implementation process, respectively. Finally, Chapter 9 describes the last two steps: framing the policy change for dissemination to the affected parties, and evaluating the effectiveness of the policy change and disseminating findings. Strategy tools are suggested for each of these steps.

Finally, Chapter 10 provides a discussion of challenges that may be encountered when engaging in evidence-informed policymaking and strategies for addressing those challenges.

Readers may note two tendencies in this book:

- At first, this book refers to evidence-*based* policymaking. But as you read, this term quickly evolves into evidence-*informed* policymaking. This is not intended as a bait and switch but rather reflects the evolution in thinking about how evidence is used in different environments. We must base clinical care on evidence, but in policymaking, the reality is that evidence merely informs.

- When we describe governmental policymaking, we primarily use the federal model as the basis for explanation. This is because it is the model for government in the US. However, much of what is accomplished in health policy actually happens at the state level—either in state legislatures or state regulatory agencies (state boards). So, those of you working at the state level, take note: You are at the epicenter of health policymaking!

It is our hope that all our readers will come away with a stronger understanding of how government works, what the policymaking process is, and how they may be able to influence policymakers to make the best use of evidence as health policies change or new health policies are introduced. Whether this influence happens at the federal or state level, in legislatures or during agency rule-making, is irrelevant; any positive influence can have an impact. For educators and students, we hope this book will help you bridge EBP and health policymaking. For those of you who are working on DNP health policy projects, we hope this book, and the EIHP model, provide process guidance. And if this book intrigues you enough to look more closely as a constituent at your own policymakers and their voting records on health policy issues, the more the better; you'll be using evidence of your own to become a more informed voter!

–Jacqueline M. Loversidge and Joyce Zurmehly

"Pretending that politics and science do not coexist is foolish, and cleanly separating science from politics is probably neither feasible nor recommended."

–Madelon Lubin Finkel

1

EXTENDING THE USE OF EVIDENCE-BASED PRACTICE TO HEALTH POLICYMAKING

–JACQUELINE M. LOVERSIDGE, PHD, RNC-AWHC

KEY CONTENT IN THIS CHAPTER

- The use of evidence in policymaking
- The evolution of evidence-based practice (EBP)
- Adapting EBP for use in health policy
- Why now is the time: reaching critical mass
- The use of research and evidence in policymaking in other countries
- The imperative for using evidence in health policymaking
- Evidence-based versus evidence-informed
- Definitions of evidence-informed policymaking

The Use of Evidence in Policymaking

Healthcare providers and consumers expect that the policies that drive, guide, and underpin healthcare will be safe and effective. Strong governmental health policy forms the foundation for healthcare funding, sustains programs for special needs groups who might otherwise find it challenging to access adequate care, and, at the state level, establishes the parameters for health professionals' scopes and standards of practice.

Nurses and other healthcare professionals involved in various professional organizations work tirelessly to advance health policy initiatives and have long mentored newcomers to their organizations who desire to do this work. Time, experience, and trial and error make for great teachers, and much of policymaking is informed by those factors. However, today's healthcare environment is so complex that trial, error, and opinion are insufficient for developing informed policy. It is therefore incumbent upon educated health professionals to press for the judicious use of science and evidence in policymaking. To do that, we must arm ourselves not only with the best evidence but with a full and realistic understanding of the political processes that are part and parcel of policymaking.

This chapter reviews the evolution of the use of evidence in the practice of medicine, in nursing and healthcare, and to inform policymaking. It presents some of the most-used evidence-based practice (EBP) models and discusses the rationale for adapting clinical practice-focused models—that is, EBP models—so they can be useful in the policymaking environment. Finally, it addresses controversies surrounding the terms *evidence-based* and *evidence-informed* and defines evidence-based policymaking.

The Evolution of Evidence-Based Practice

Historically, good conventional medical practice was based on tradition, and clinical measures considered to be successful were passed on from mentor to student. This unquestioned practice of treating patients based on an oral tradition of unknown or forgotten origin began to change in the late Middle Ages, when physician-scholars—often men of the cloth—took on the practice of medicine. These healers focused on gaining a new understanding of past thought and practice through the exploration of natural science and experimentation and the search for medical truth (Daly & Brater, 2000). Historians believe the early foundations of evidence-based medicine were laid in the 17th and 18th centuries—a positive effect of the Enlightenment, as medicine turned toward the evaluation and interpretation of scientific evidence (Gerber, Lungen, & Lauterbach, 2005). The use of EBP, as we have come to know it, grew out of this long, slow evolution toward EBM.

Evidence-Based Medicine to Evidence-Based Practice

As the conduct of research in medicine evolved, practice developed and changed in response, keeping pace with the available science. But as this conduct of research became more sophisticated and the practice of medicine matured, physicians realized that findings from a single study—no matter how robust—were insufficient to ethically justify sweeping change in practice. Accordingly, practitioners sought to integrate a body of work culled from the best research findings into their practice.

In addition to the problems associated with insufficient evidence, the time it takes to conduct research and the lag between publication of research and adoption of the knowledge gleaned by that research into practice also became apparent. Incredibly, the average time lag in the health research translation process is 17 years (Morris, Wooding, & Grant, 2011). To improve this process, the field of translation science developed. Titler (2014) defines *translation science* as "a field of research that focuses on testing implementation interventions to improve uptake and use of evidence to improve patient outcomes and population health, and to explicate what implementation strategies work for whom, in what settings, and why" (p. 270).

Time and experience yielded valuable lessons about how to translate findings from research into practice. But science, isolated from the realities of practice, could not serve the needs of both practitioners and patients. Human factors needed to be considered, including clinician experience and judgment, as well as the patient's lived experience, values, and healthcare objectives. As a result, a process that integrated scientific findings, the patient's needs, and the practitioner's expertise was developed by physicians for use in medicine. It was, and is still, called *evidence-based medicine* (EBM).

As EBM evolved, its definition included reference to the conscientious use of current best evidence for making decisions about patient care (Sackett, Straus,

Richardson, Rosenberg, & Haynes, 2000). An updated and well-accepted definition is: "Evidence-based medicine (EBM) requires the integration of the best research evidence with our clinical expertise and our patient's unique values and circumstances" (Straus, Richardson, Glasziou, & Haynes, 2011, p. 1).

The term *EBM* is self-limited because it refers only to the practice of medicine. Consequently, other health professions sought to broaden the definition and embraced the more inclusive term *practice*. The term *evidence-based practice* is now widely used among non-physician healthcare providers. More than 50 models of EBP have emerged in the literature to address the needs of nursing practice, education, and science; one EBP model is transdisciplinary (Satterfield et al., 2009; Stevens, 2013).

Evidence-Based Practice Models

EBP models share a common purpose, regardless of the differences in their processes and structures: They establish a systematic method for the user to ask clinical questions, search for and synthesize evidence, and translate what is found in the research to be serviceable in practice settings. All EBP models are process models. They largely aim to assist the process of clinical decision-making to improve patient-care quality and outcomes (Mitchell, Fisher, Hastings, Silverman, & Wallen, 2010).

Definitions of EBP are model-dependent but generally take a three-pronged or three-legged stool approach. An established definition of EBP is:

> a paradigm and lifelong problem-solving approach to clinical decision making that involves the conscientious use of the best available evidence . . . with one's own clinical expertise and patient values and preferences to improve outcomes for individuals, groups, communities, and systems. (Melnyk & Fineout-Overholt, 2015, p. 604)

Although there are numerous types of EBP models, six nursing EBP models are selected for description here, as they are some of the most frequently discussed in the literature. These models are as follows:

- The Academic Center for Evidence-Based Practice (ACE) Star Model of Knowledge Transformation

- The Advancing Research and Clinical Practice Through Close Collaboration (ARCC) Model
- The Iowa Model
- The Johns Hopkins Nursing EBP (JHNEBP) Model
- The Promoting Action on Research Implementation in Health Services (PARIHS) Framework
- The Stetler Model

These EBP models demonstrate commonalities in their purpose, but their unique attributes make them more or less useful for organizations or individual healthcare providers, with some models being useful for both. Organizations, individual healthcare providers, and healthcare educators can choose which model to use based on the intended purpose and best fit. Summaries and overviews of the predominant EBP models have been published (Dang et. al., 2015; Schaffer, Sandau, & Diedrick, 2013); brief overviews of model and framework elements are provided here.

The Academic Center for Evidence-Based Practice (ACE) Star Model of Knowledge Transformation

This model is designed for use by either organizations or individual providers. It focuses on locating nursing evidence for practice at the bedside and addresses ways to effect the adoption of innovation. Key steps of the model are as follows (Kring, 2008; Stevens, 2013; The University of Texas Health Science Center School of Nursing, 2015):

1. Discovery
2. Evidence summary
3. Translation
4. Integration
5. Evaluation

The Advancing Research and Clinical Practice Through Close Collaboration (ARCC) Model

This model, developed by Melnyk, Fineout-Overholt, Gallagher-Ford, & Stillwell (2011), takes organizational culture and readiness into account and is an ideal fit for use in large organizations (Schaffer et al., 2013). The ARCC Model is based on the following assumptions:

- Healthcare systems have both barriers to and facilitators for EBP implementation.
- For individuals or systems to implement EBP, barriers must be removed or minimized, and facilitators mounted or strengthened.
- Clinicians must develop belief in EBP and confidence in their ability to carry out EBP.
- Successful advancement of a systemic EBP culture requires mentors.

Steps in the ARCC Model begin with an assessment of organizational culture and readiness for the implementation of EBP system-wide, proceed to an identification of the strengths of and barriers to EBP, and move to the development and use of EBP mentors in the organization (Melnyk et al., 2011). The ARCC Model has been widely used and tested, and valid, reliable instruments are available for measuring its key constructs (Dang et al., 2015).

The Iowa Model

The emphasis of the Iowa Model is on its use in an organization. It is particularly applicable in interdisciplinary settings. This model features a team approach and focuses on the identification of practice questions, the search for and critique or synthesis of evidence, and problem-solving steps including pilot testing of selected EBP changes. A flowchart guides organizational decision-making, and feedback loops are helpful for determining when a change in direction is needed. For example, is there sufficient research to pilot a practice change? If not, then one should base practice on other types of evidence or conduct additional research. Essential steps in the model are as follows (Schaffer et al., 2013; Titler et al., 2001):

1. Identify practice questions.
2. Determine whether the topic is an organizational priority.
3. Form a team to search for, critique, and synthesize evidence.
4. Determine evidence sufficiency.
5. Pilot the change if evidence is sufficient.
6. Evaluate the pilot, disseminate results, and, if successful, implement the program into practice.

The Johns Hopkins Nursing EBP (JHNEBP) Model

The Johns Hopkins Nursing EBP (JHNEBP) Model is a practical model designed for use by bedside nurses. The model emphasizes the identification of the practice question and the skilled evaluation of evidence. Attention is given to the translation of research to practice. The construction of an implementation plan is also an important model element. The three-step model is called PET, short for practice question, evidence, and translation. These steps are summarized as follows (Dang et al., 2015; Johns Hopkins Medicine, n.d.; Schaffer et al., 2013):

1. Identify the practice question (the EBP question) using a team approach.

2. Search for, critique, and summarize the evidence, and develop strong, feasible recommendations accordingly.

3. Translate the recommendations by moving them into an actionable practice change that is implemented, evaluated, and communicated.

The Promoting Action on Research Implementation in Health Services (PARIHS) Framework

The Promoting Action on Research Implementation in Health Services (PARIHS) Framework includes core elements of evidence, context, and facilitation as a framework for the practice change process. The framework highlights the impact of context on EBP success—for example, leadership support (Schaffer et al., 2013). The framework has been developed and refined, applied in a variety of settings, and complements other EBP models. It has also been developed to recognize and make best use of organizational complexity. The model uses a dynamic framework consisting of elements and multiple sub-elements. The major elements are evidence, context, and facilitation (Dang et al., 2015). Revisions to the framework, with accompanying tools for implementation, have been made available (Dang et al., 2015; Stetler, Damschroder, Helfrich, & Hagedorn, 2011).

The Stetler Model

The Stetler Model was originally developed with a focus on research utilization but has been updated to merge conceptually with the EBP paradigm. The model is individual provider-focused but can be useful for promoting organizational change toward the use of EBP in that it gives explicit support for individuals working in groups responsible for advancing practice change (Stetler, 2001). Its emphasis is on critical thinking. Like the PARIHS Framework, it also acknowledges the importance of context for advancing EBP (Schaffer et al., 2013).

Applying EBP Models to Practice

Each of the EBP models described provides effective processes for addressing complex clinical problems. Whether the model is designed for use by individual providers or organizations, each model requires that the user do each of the following:

1. Ask a clinical question.
2. Search the literature to identify a body of evidence.
3. Use a systematic process to critique and synthesize the evidence.
4. Take logical steps to determine whether the body of evidence is sufficient to support a practice change.

Healthcare systems are urged to integrate EBP into their organizational cultures as a means to improve patient outcomes and reduce cost. To do so, registered nurses (RNs) and advance practice registered nurses (APRNs) alike have been called upon to develop expertise in EBP. To achieve this, EBP competencies specific for RNs and APRNs have been developed; it is now imperative that healthcare systems commit to a plan that integrates these competencies into the practice culture so that an EBP-competent nursing workforce becomes the standard. Leadership support and EBP mentorship are essential components of any system meant to promote EBP in an organization (Melnyk, Fineout-Overholt, Giggleman, & Choy, 2017; Melnyk, Gallagher-Ford, Long, & Fineout-Overholt, 2014).

Adapting EBP for Use in Health Policy

Policy-related frameworks and models are useful for strategizing to advance a health policy agenda and for analyzing existing or pending health policy. These are addressed in detail in Chapter 5, "Policymaking Processes and Models." However, as nurses and other health professionals are gaining competency in EBP, it is a natural extension for them to draw upon their understanding of EBP models to address health policy problems.

Clearly, a number of excellent EBP models exist. All these models use evidence to solve problems and are designed to be useful in complex environments. Because of these attributes, EBP models lend themselves to use in the health policy milieu, if they are modified. There are two primary reasons why EBP models are particularly adaptable to health policymaking:

- Although EBP models are designed to address clinical issues, they are predominantly process models. As such, the approaches suggested in EBP models for identifying and describing problems, searching the literature, appraising and synthesizing evidence, and taking steps to determine the best path to accomplish a practice change are similar to those needed to address health policy issues (Loversidge, 2016a).

- In addition to research evidence, EBP models consider factors such as internal evidence, clinician expertise, patient values and preferences, and mentor or organizational support and facilitation (Melnyk & Fineout-Overholt, 2015; Schaffer et al., 2013). The consideration of these additional factors enables EBP models to adapt particularly well to complex policy environments (Loversidge, 2016a).

There are, however, significant differences between clinical organization environments and the policymaking environment, which necessitate the adaptation of EBP models for this alternate use. Most notably, in most clinical environments, providers from across clinical disciplines and leadership agree on the mission: to serve the patient's health and safety needs, improve outcomes, and lower costs. This kind of singular focus is rarely seen in policymaking, however. Government policy priorities are established by a commander-in-chief—that is, the president of the United States or the state governor—as well as by the majority party. Therefore, partisan politics necessarily become a part of the agenda-setting formula.

In addition, priority timelines shift according to the time of year and the legislative cycle. For example, during the budget cycle, attention is focused on the budget bill. Similarly, at the end of a two-year congressional or legislative session, bills that are favored politically and considered a priority will be pushed to passage, while bills that aren't are likely to languish and die.

Add to that the fact that stakeholders—and their interests in legislation—are numerous and varied. Lobbyists representing professional associations or business organizations, private citizens or consumers, individual professionals, and a host of others seek to influence the outcome of the policymaking process. Some factors and relationships are flexible, in which case the potential to sway opposition by building relationships, reaching compromise, or influencing a legislator's vote may or may not present itself. Other factors are immovable, such as the timing of budget cycles, legislative sessions, and election seasons.

Because of these factors, the direct application of clinical EBP models to the policymaking process would be, at best, difficult and awkward. The language of EBP is not a direct fit for policymaking, the stakeholders are different and more varied, and the policymaking processes do not occur in an orderly fashion. Policymaking is necessarily a messy and nonlinear process; it's often a case of two steps forward and three steps back. Therefore, although EBP models and frameworks provide, in concept, an ideal foundation for preparing nurses and healthcare providers to use evidence in policymaking, these models must be adapted to be useful in the policymaking process.

Why Now Is the Time: Reaching Critical Mass

One persuasive reason to advance the utilization of EBP in health policymaking is that nurses are becoming increasingly familiar with, and gaining competency in, EBP. Although there is much room for the growth of competency in this area, more nurses are EBP-competent now than ever before (Melnyk & Fineout-Overholt, 2015; Melnyk et al., 2014). Other healthcare providers are also becoming more familiar with EBP processes.

Nurses and other healthcare providers are less accustomed to health policymaking, so the use of a recognizable model to approach policy problems can provide both a sense of comfort and a sense of mastery. Nurses across the practice and leadership spectrum—RNs, APRNs, nurse managers and chief nursing officers, nurses in leadership and advocacy positions in professional associations, and so on—are becoming familiar with the use of EBP as a process to resolve clinical problems. In addition, nursing educators are called on to teach EBP to students at both the undergraduate and the graduate levels (American Association of Colleges of Nursing [AACN], 2006; AACN, 2008; AACN, 2011), providing a measure of assurance that the next cadre of nursing professionals will have a level of EBP competency.

The nursing profession is approaching a critical mass of EBP-competent nurses who will be able to advance the use of EBP in health policymaking (Loversidge, 2016a). Concurrently, the nursing profession has put out the call for nurses to advance the health of the nation by serving on boards and making changes at the policy level (Institute of Medicine [IOM], 2010). A nonexhaustive list of national nursing policy and advocacy priorities that could be facilitated by an evidence-based approach includes the following (AACN, 2018; American Association of Nurse Practitioners, 2018; American Nurses Association, 2018; National League for Nursing, 2017):

- Safe staffing
- Workplace health and safety
- Supporting operable information technology
- Protecting and improving provisions of the Affordable Care Act
- Accessibility, affordability, diversity, excellence, and efficiency in higher education for nurses
- Improved funding, efficiency, and safety for biomedical and health-care research
- Focus on value-based models of person-centered, prevention-focused care
- Licensure/state practice environments and access to care

The Use of Research and Evidence in Policymaking in Other Countries

The US has trailed European countries and Canada in its use of evidence in policymaking. The United Kingdom, the Netherlands, and Canada were early adopters, having used evidence in the development of health policy for almost 20 years (Dobrow, Goel, & Upshur, 2004; Elliott & Popay, 2000; Niessen, Grijseels, & Rutten, 2000). The literature is rich with examples from other countries.

At the turn of the millennium, a group of researchers from the Netherlands explored and reported on evidence-based approaches in health policy and healthcare delivery at three levels of impact (Niessen et al., 2000):

- Intersectoral assessment with or without collaboration of the health sector

- National healthcare policy

- Evidence-based medicine

Their analysis predicted a growing demand for *intersectoral assessment,* which is assessment undertaken by actors outside the health sector. Additionally, they found that governments were largely increasing their support for and use of evidence in health policymaking and that EBP and treatment guidelines published by independent professional organizations were gaining prominence.

Concurrently, researchers from the UK conducted a qualitative study to better understand the influence of evidence on policymakers within the UK's National Health Service (NHS) after a period of NHS reform. Whereas in medicine and in the health science professions, the effect of evidence on quality improvement is fairly direct, these policy researchers found that the effect of evidence on policymakers was more indirect. They discovered that research was more likely to affect and mediate the policy debate or to be used in dialogue between stakeholders. They also found that when policymakers made decisions, their knowledge and experience, budget limitations, and time constraints countered even the strongest evidence. The researchers noted, however, that sustained dialogue between policymakers and researchers improved utilization of evidence in the policymaking process (Elliott & Popay, 2000).

The importance of separating individual clinical decision-making from evidence-based decision-making at a population-policy level was studied by collaborating researchers from the UK and Canada. They noted that decision-making at the policy level is rife with uncertainty, variability, and complexity. They also observed that in health policymaking, the use of evidence may be more important than how it is defined. From this research they developed an evidence-utilization process model as a basis for a context-based conceptual framework of evidence-based decision-making in health policy (Dobrow et al., 2004).

The US has gained momentum in its use of evidence in policymaking. This is in part a result of the groundswell of health policy experts and healthcare professionals who have interest and expertise in compiling relevant evidence to help policymakers with their work. However, an additional force for change was initiated during the Obama administration: Public Law 114-140, which was passed by the US Congress to create the Commission on Evidence-Based Policymaking. The commission's report was released September 7, 2017, and its recommendations heard during a meeting of the full House Committee on Oversight and Government Reform on September 26, 2017. Chapter 2, "Using Evidence: The Changing Landscape in Health Policymaking," provides a summary of that report and a discussion of two companion bills subsequently introduced in the US House and Senate.

The Imperative for Using Evidence in Health Policymaking

Some say that the term *evidence-based policymaking* is an oxymoron. Even though the social and economic realities that account for many of our nation's negative health outcomes are amenable to improvement through health policy reform, policy changes are driven largely by ideology and bias instead of evidence (Fishbeyn, 2015). Still, the potential for positive change in the nation's policy through the use of evidence is promising, as long as the complexity of the policymaking process is understood, appreciated, and leveraged.

Leaders in nursing, nursing education, and nursing regulation have made significant contributions to the advancement of evidence-based policymaking. Numerous nursing health policy textbooks include the role of research and EBP applications in health policymaking. The National Council of State Boards of Nursing and leaders from state boards of nursing tirelessly advance evidence-based policymaking in regulation (Damgaard & Young, 2017; National Council of State Boards of Nursing Practice, Regulation and Education Committee, 2006; Ridenour, 2009; Spector, 2010). And our nation's nursing leaders have long advocated for change in how nurses contribute to health policymaking (IOM, 2010).

EBP models, adapted for use in health policymaking, are useful tools for actors who intend to influence policymakers. They are especially important, however, for individuals who serve in leadership positions in nursing and other health profession associations or health-related government agencies. Those who work in government agencies have a more formal role in policymaking, so using a solid evidence base to influence policymakers and stakeholders is essential. Using an evidence-based health policy model that considers context and stakeholders in addition to evidence allows for a more logical and complete analysis of the policymaking environment and permits a more realistic strategy to emerge.

Nurse educators can use an evidence-based health policymaking model to teach students about health policy. Using the steps of an evidence-based policymaking process can help students gain an understanding of the overall health policymaking process, analyze and understand health policy issues more completely, and formulate strategies to effect change. Students can apply the steps of the process to pending or existing policy or use the process to strategically plan their own policy response to a known health policy problem.

Evidence-Based Versus Evidence-Informed

At the turn of the millennium, health policy scientists became familiar with the use of research to inform policymaking. They had become accustomed to the use of both single studies and systematic reviews as sources of evidence but were coming around to the idea that these sources alone were insufficient for informing policy discussions with legislators. They reached consensus that a more extensive body of evidence was required. As a result, the term *evidence-based* came into use in policymaking (Dobrow et al., 2004; Niessen et al., 2000; Pawson, 2006).

Around the same time that EBP emerged as a complement to EBM in the health professions, the term *evidence-based* was established as the norm in policymaking. However, policy leaders and scientists noted that there is often a considerable gap between the scientific evidence presented to policymakers and a policy as it is enacted (Brownson, Chriqui, & Stamatakis, 2009). Consequently, these leaders and scientists began to lean toward the term *evidence-informed* rather than *evidence-based* because it is a more accurate reflection of the realities and complexities of the policy environment.

The term *evidence-informed* is useful and important in policymaking for several reasons:

- **It acknowledges the boundaries of the use of evidence in policymaking:** As discussed, in policymaking, the use of evidence has been found to be indirect. Its best uses are to inform, mediate, or influence dialogue between stakeholders (Campbell et al., 2009; Elliott & Popay, 2000; Lavis et al., 2009; Morgan, 2010). Stakeholders may consist of individuals or groups including lawmakers, lobbyists, service providers, consumers, and other professionals.

- **It recognizes the rapidly changing, politically charged policy environment:** Limited budgets, budget cycles, and the timing of congressional or legislative sessions are inflexible and affect both priorities and stakeholder relationships (Bowen & Zwi, 2005; Jewell & Bero, 2008).

- **It acknowledges a global standard that has emerged for health policy over the past decade:** The term *evidence-informed* pressed itself into use when the World Health Organization (WHO) EVIPNet Knowledge Translation Platform (KTP) was established in 2005. The WHO EVIPNet KTP has advanced the systematic use of evidence in health policymaking since that time and is known as the *Evidence-Informed Policy Network* (WHO, 2018). In 2009, the journal *Health Research Policy and Systems* solidified use of the term by publishing a supplemental issue that provided support tools for evidence-informed health policymaking (Lavis et al., 2009).

Definitions of Evidence-Informed Policymaking

A variety of definitions of evidence-informed policymaking exist. There are common themes among them; what distinguishes the definitions is their source and purpose.

This section provides five definitions of evidence-informed policymaking. The first two originate from health policy-focused sources. The next two are not directly health-focused but are helpful in that one is in plain language, while the other shows the level of detail necessitated by government policy reports.

The fifth is a definition for evidence-informed health policy for use in nursing education and regulation, which may be extended to general healthcare policymaking.

The first definition underpins the SUPPORT tools for evidence-informed health policymaking (Oxman, Lavis, Lewin, & Fretheim, 2009). The SUPPORT project, initiated by the European Commission, generated a series of articles for individuals responsible for making health policy and program decisions. The SUPPORT definition follows:

> Evidence-informed health policymaking is an approach to policy decisions that aims to ensure that decision making is well-informed by the best available research evidence. It is characterized by the systematic and transparent access to, and appraisal of, evidence as an input into the policymaking process. (Oxman et al., 2009, p. 1)

The second definition comes from the WHO EVIPNet, which speaks to "promot[ing] the systematic use of research evidence in health policymaking in order to strengthen health systems and get the right programs, services and drugs to those who need them" (2018).

The Overseas Development Institute (ODI) is the source of the third definition. The ODI is an independent think tank that promotes global progress by focusing on research and analysis to develop sustainable solutions for significant problems. Its definition of evidence-informed policymaking is "when policymakers use the best available evidence to help make policy decisions . . . [this includes] scientific research . . . [and also] statistical data, citizen voice, and evaluation evidence" (Ball, 2018).

The fourth definition comes from the Commission on Evidence-Based Policymaking (2017). Its definition focuses on the meanings of the word *evidence* rather than on a process:

> "Evidence" can be defined broadly as information that aids the generation of a conclusion . . . this report uses the shorthand "evidence" to refer to information produced by "statistical activities" with a "statistical purpose" that is potentially useful when evaluating government programs and policies . . . we define "statistical activities" as "the collection, compilation, processing, analysis, or dissemination of data for the purpose of describing or making

estimates concerning the whole, or relevant groups or components within, the economy, society, or the natural environment, including the development of methods or resources that support those activities, such as measurement of methods, statistical classifications, or sampling frames." A "statistical purpose" is defined as "the description, estimation, or analysis of the characteristics of groups . . . and includes the development, implementation, or maintenance of methods, technical or administrative procedures, or information resources that support such purposes." (pp. 8–11)

The last definition comes from the evidence-informed health policy (EIHP) model used throughout much of this text. It is an adaptation of the Melnyk and Fineout-Overholt definition of EBP (2015). In the EIHP model, evidence-informed health policy "combines the use of the best available evidence and issue expertise with stakeholder values and ethics to inform and leverage dialogue toward the best possible health policy agenda and improvements" (Loversidge, 2016b).

Summary

This chapter discussed why evidence should be considered in health policymaking. It began by explaining how EBP evolved from EBM. EBP is a process that addresses clinical problems and improves the quality of healthcare and patient outcomes. A number of nursing-specific EBP models exist; this chapter offered a non-exhaustive list of those models and described them in brief. All of these are process models and therefore may be adapted to non-clinical, health-related problems, including health policy problems.

The chapter went on to note that evidence-based policymaking has been advanced in other countries, particularly in Western Europe and Canada, and is now gaining traction in the US. It explained why nurses and other health professionals who have competency in EBP are positioned to adapt these skills. Finally, it discussed how evidence-based or evidence-informed policymaking can address health policy problems and help nurses and other healthcare providers influence, inform, and advance positive change in health policy.

References

American Association of Colleges of Nursing. (2006). *The essentials of doctoral education for advanced nursing practice.* Retrieved from https://www.aacnnursing.org/Portals/42/Publications/DNPEssentials.pdf

American Association of Colleges of Nursing. (2008*). The essentials of baccalaureate education for professional nursing practice.* Retrieved from https://www.aacnnursing.org/Portals/42/Publications/BaccEssentials08.pdf

American Association of Colleges of Nursing. (2011). *The essentials of master's education in nursing.* Retrieved from https://www.aacnnursing.org/Portals/42/Publications/MastersEssentials11.pdf

American Association of Colleges of Nursing. (2018). Federal policy agenda 2017–2018. Retrieved from https://www.aacnnursing.org/Policy-Advocacy/About-Government-Affairs-and-Policy/Federal-Policy-Agenda

American Association of Nurse Practitioners. (2018). Legislation/regulation. Retrieved from https://www.aanp.org/legislation-regulation

American Nurses Association (2018*).* Legislative and regulatory priorities for the 115th Congress. Retrieved from https://www.nursingworld.org/practice-policy/advocacy/federal/115-congress-legislative-and-regulatory-priorities/

Ball, Louise. (2018, Jan. 2). Explainer: What is evidence-informed policymaking? *Overseas Development Institute.* Retrieved from https://www.odi.org/comment/10592-explainer-what-evidence-informed-policy-making

Bowen, S., & Zwi, A. B. (2005). Pathways to "evidence-informed" policy and practice: A framework for action. *PLoS Medicine, 2*(7), e166.

Brownson, R. C., Chriqui, J. F., & Stamatakis, K. A. (2009). Understanding evidence-based public health policy. *American Journal of Public Health, 99*(9), 1576–1583. doi:10.2105/AJPH.2008.156224

Campbell, D. M., Redman, S., Jorm, L., Cooke, M., Zwi, A. B., & Rychetnik, L. (2009). Increasing the use of evidence in health policy: Practice and views of policy makers and researchers. *Australia & New Zealand Health Policy, 6,* 21. doi:10.1186/1743-8462-6-21

Commission on Evidence-Based Policymaking. (2017). *The promise of evidence-based policymaking.* Retrieved from https://www.cep.gov/content/dam/cep/report/cep-final-report.pdf

Daly, W. J., and Brater, D. C. (2000). Medieval contributions to the search for truth in clinical medicine. *Perspectives in Biology and Medicine, 43*(4), 530–540.

Damgaard, G., & Young, L. (2017) Application of an evidence-informed health policy model for the decision to delegate insulin administration. *Journal of Nursing Regulation, 7*(4), 33–40.

Dang, D., Melnyk, B. M., Fineout-Overhold, E., Ciliska, D., DiCenso, A., Cullen, L., . . . Stevens, K. R. (2015). Models to guide implementation and sustainability of evidence-based practice. In B. M. Melnyk & E. Fineout-Overholt (Eds.), *Evidence-based practice in nursing & healthcare: A guide to practice* (3rd ed., pp. 274–315). Philadelphia, PA: Lippincott Williams & Wilkins.

Dobrow, M. J., Goel, V., & Upshur, R. E. (2004). Evidence-based health policy: Context and utilisation. *Social Science & Medicine, 58*(1), 207–217.

Elliott, H., & Popay, J. (2000). How are policy makers using evidence? Models of research utilisation and local NHS policy making. *Journal of Epidemiology & Community Health, 54*(6), 461–468.

Fishbeyn, B. (2015). When ideology trumps: A case for evidence-based health policies. *The American Journal of Bioethics, 15*(3), 1–2. doi:10:10.1080/15265161.2015.1019781

Gerber, A., Lungen, M., & Lauterbach, K. W. (2005). Evidence-based medicine is rooted in the Protestant exegesis. *Medical Hypotheses, 64*(5), 1034–1038.

Institute of Medicine. (2010). *The future of nursing: Leading change, advancing health.* Washington, DC: The National Academies Press.

Jewell, C. J., & Bero, L. A. (2008). "Developing good taste in evidence": Facilitators of and hindrances to evidence-informed health policymaking in state government. *The Milbank Quarterly, 86*(2), 177–208.

Johns Hopkins Medicine. (n.d.). Center for Evidence-Based Practice. Retrieved from https://www.hopkinsmedicine.org/evidence-based-practice/ijhn_2017_ebp.html

Kring, D. L. (2008). Clinical nurse specialist practice domains and evidence-based practice competencies: A matrix of influence. *Clinical Nurse Specialist, 22*(4), 179–183.

Lavis, J. N., Oxman, A. D., Souza, N. M., Lewin, S., Gruen, R. L., & Fretheim, A. (2009). SUPPORT tools for evidence-informed health policymaking (STP) 9: Assessing the applicability of the findings of a systematic review. *Health Research Policy and Systems, 7* (Suppl. 1), 1–7.

Loversidge, J. M. (2016a). A call for extending the utility of evidence-based practice: Adapting EBP for health policy impact. *Worldviews on Evidence-Based Nursing, 13*(6), 399–401. doi:10.1111/wvn.12183

Loversidge, J. M. (2016b). An evidence-informed health policy model: Adapting evidence-based practice for nursing education and regulation. *Journal of Nursing Regulation, 7*(2), 27–33.

Melnyk, B. M., & Fineout-Overholt, E. (2015). *Evidence-based practice in nursing and healthcare: A guide to best practice* (3rd ed.). Philadelphia, PA: Lippincott Williams & Wilkins.

Melnyk, B. M., Fineout-Overholt, E., Gallagher-Ford, L., & Stillwell, S. B. (2011). Evidence-based practice, step by step: Sustaining evidence-based practice through organizational policies and an innovative model. *American Journal of Nursing, 111*(9), 57–60.

Melnyk, B. M., Fineout-Overholt, E., Giggleman, M., & Choy, K. (2017). A test of the ARCC model improves implementation of evidence-based practice, healthcare culture, and patient outcomes. *Worldviews on Evidence-Based Nursing, 14*(1), 5–9.

Melnyk, B. M., Gallagher-Ford, L., Long, L. E., & Fineout-Overholt, E. (2014). The establishment of evidence-based practice competencies for practicing nurses and advanced practice nurses in real-world clinical settings: Proficiencies to improve healthcare quality, reliability, patient outcomes, and costs. *Worldviews on Evidence-Based Nursing, 11*(1), 5–15.

Mitchell, S. A., Fisher, C. A., Hastings, C. E., Silverman, L. B., & Wallen, G. R. (2010). A thematic analysis of theoretical models for translational science in nursing: Mapping the field. *Nursing Outlook, 58*(6), 287–300. doi:10.1016/j.outlook.2010.07.001

Morgan, G. (2010). Evidence-based health policy: A preliminary systematic review. *Health Education Journal, 69*(1), 43–47. doi:10.1177/0017896910363328

Morris, Z. S., Wooding, S., & Grant, J. (2011). The answer is 17 years, what is the question: Understanding time lags in translational research. *Journal of the Royal Society of Medicine, 104*(12), 510–520. doi:10.1258/jrsm.2011.110180

National Council of State Boards of Nursing Practice, Regulation and Education Committee. (2006). Evidence-based nursing education for regulation (EBNER). Retrieved from https://www.ncsbn.org/Final_06_EBNER_Report.pdf

National League for Nursing. (2017). *Public policy agenda 2017–2018*. Retrieved from http://www.nln.org/docs/default-source/advocacy-public-policy/public-policy-agenda-pdf.pdf?sfvrsn=2

Niessen, L. W., Grijseels, E. W., & Rutten, F. F. (2000). The evidence-based approach in health policy and health care delivery. *Social Science & Medicine, 51*(6), 859–869.

Oxman, A. D., Lavis, J. N., Lewin, S., & Fretheim, A. (2009). SUPPORT tools for evidence-informed health policymaking (STP) 1: What is evidence-informed policymaking? *Health Research Policy and Systems, 7*(Suppl. 1), S1. doi:10.1 186/1478-4505-7-S1-S1

Pawson, R. (2006). Evidence-based policy: The promise of a systematic review. In R. Pawson (Ed.), *Evidence-based policy: A realist perspective* (pp. 2–17). London, UK: Sage Publications Ltd. doi:10.4135/9781849209120.n1

Ridenour, J. (2009). Evidence-based regulation: Emerging knowledge management to inform policy. In K. Malloch & T. Porter-O'Grady (Eds.), *Introduction to evidence-based practice in nursing and health care*. (pp. 275–299). Sudbury, MA: Jones and Bartlett Learning.

Sackett, D. L., Straus, S. E., Richardson, W. S., Rosenberg, W., & Haynes, R. B. (2000). *Evidence-based medicine: How to practice and teach EBM* (2nd ed.). London, UK: Churchill Livingstone Elsevier.

Satterfield, J. M., Spring, B., Brownson, R. C., Mullen, E. J., Newhouse, R. P., Walker, B. B., & Whitlock, E. P. (2009). Toward a transdisciplinary model of evidence-based practice. *The Milbank Quarterly, 87*(2), 368–390.

Schaffer, M. A., Sandau, K. E., & Diedrick, L. (2013). Evidence-based practice models for organizational change: Overview and practical applications. *Journal of Advanced Nursing, 69*(5), 1197–1209. doi:10.1111/j.1365-2648.2012.06122.x

Spector, N. (2010). Evidence-based nursing regulation: A challenge for regulators. *Journal of Nursing Regulation, 1*(1), 30–36.

Stetler, C. B. (2001). Updating the Stetler Model of research utilization to facilitate evidence-based practice. *Nursing Outlook, 49*(6), 272–279.

Stetler, C. B., Damschroder, L. J., Helfrich, C. D., and Hagedorn, H. J. (2011). A guide for applying a revised version of the PARIHS framework for implementation. *Implementation Science, 6*, 99–109.

Stevens, K. R. (2013). The impact of evidence-based practice in nursing and the next big ideas. *Online Journal of Issues in Nursing, 18*(2), Manuscript 4. doi:10.3912/OJIN.Vol18No02Man04

Straus, S. E., Richardson, W. S., Glasziou, P., & Haynes, R. B. (2011). *Evidence-based medicine: How to practice and teach it* (4th ed.). London, UK: Churchill Livingstone Elsevier.

Titler, M. G. (2014). Overview of evidence-based practice and translation science. *The Nursing Clinics of North America, 49*(3), 269–274.

Titler, M. G., Kleiber, C., Steelman, V., Rakel, B. A., Budreau, G., Everett, L. Q., . . . Goode, C. (2001). The Iowa Model of evidence-based practice to promote quality care. *Critical Care Nursing Clinics of North America, 13*(4), 497–509.

The University of Texas Health Science Center School of Nursing. (2015). Star Model. Retrieved from http://nursing.uthscsa.edu/onrs/starmodel/star-model.asp

World Health Organization. (2018). Evidence-Informed Policy Network: What is EVIPNet? Retrieved from http://www.who.int/evidence/about/en/

"Change will not come if we wait for some other person or if we wait for some other time. We are the ones we've been waiting for. We are the change that we seek."

–Barack Obama

2

USING EVIDENCE: THE CHANGING LANDSCAPE IN HEALTH POLICYMAKING

–JACQUELINE M. LOVERSIDGE, PHD, RNC-AWHC

KEY CONTENT IN THIS CHAPTER

- The emerging and controversial uses of science, research, and evidence in policymaking
- Sources of guidance for evaluating evidence to inform policymaking
- Examples of the use and influence of evidence on policy-making and practice
- The changing perspectives on the use of evidence and of "big data"
- Strategies for using evidence in policymaking for nurses and other healthcare professionals

The Emerging and Controversial Uses of Science, Research, and Evidence in Policymaking

Chapter 1, "Extending the Use of Evidence-Based Practice to Health Policy-making," introduced the concept of evidence-based or evidence-*informed* policymaking and its steady (if uneven) adoption in the United States and other countries. The consensus is that the appropriate use of evidence—particularly scientific evidence—will improve and legitimize the policy decision-making process (Montuschi, 2009). Hence, over the past 20 years, emphasis has been placed on using evidence to nudge government policy programming toward higher performance and greater accountability (Hall & Jennings, 2010; Maynard, 2006).

Later chapters address the process of searching for and collecting the most relevant and best evidence to inform health policymaking and using an evidence-informed policymaking model. First, however, it is important to consider what constitutes evidence and how it is used in policymaking. That is what this chapter is about.

Context for Evidence in Policymaking

Context is essential in policymaking. It is therefore an important consideration when it comes to the use of evidence.

The context for evidence in policymaking is different from that of evidence-based medicine (EBM) or evidence-based practice (EBP) because of the nature of the policymaking environment. Scientists and healthcare providers largely look at evidence as scientific and usually attach greater importance to evidence that can be viewed as objective and context-free. The scientific view of evidence is that it is information that has been generated through a prescribed process. This process yields information or facts that are explicit, that have been systematically obtained using clear and transparent methods, and that are replicable—in other words, researchers following the same methods can attain the same results, or results that are otherwise observable, credible, verifiable, or supportable (Lomas, Culyer, McCutcheon, McAuley, & Law, 2005).

In policymaking, the scientific view of evidence might be useful depending on the substance of the policy being considered. However, context-sensitive evidence may be just as useful or even more so. In contrast to scientific evidence, context-based evidence, called *colloquial evidence,* establishes facts or gives reason to believe in something.

When evidence is defined as colloquial, its test of inclusion is more personal and normally depends on local relevance rather than methodological testing (Lomas et al., 2005). For example, in the healthcare sciences and professions, it is important to know whether a drug, diagnostic tool, or intervention will work, and on which populations. In policymaking, it is equally important to know whether a policy is *likely* to work and whether advancing the policy will be worth the effort and expenditure of political capital.

In policymaking, evidence is gathered to ensure that the best available research is used as one input into the policymaking process. This process is not always systematic, linear, or transparent. As a part of the overall process, policymakers should consider a systematic procedure for identifying, appraising, and using the best available research to help policymakers understand the issues and potential policy solutions (Oxman, Lavis, Lewin, & Fretheim, 2009). Both scientific and colloquial evidence must be considered, however.

Evidence and Evidence Hierarchies: What Constitutes Evidence in Health Policy?

The quality of an evidence source, how evidence is summarized and interpreted, and how it is used matter as much in policymaking as those considerations do in clinical decision-making. Therefore, understanding what may constitute evidence appropriate for health policymaking is as important as appreciating the differences in how evidence is used in policymaking and clinical decision-making.

Simply put, in policymaking, evidence is understood to concern facts—actual or asserted—intended to support a conclusion (Lomas et al., 2005). It is important to understand that "evidence can be used to support a conclusion, but it is not the same as a conclusion. Evidence alone does not make decisions" (Oxman et al., 2009, p. 3).

To illustrate which pieces of evidence are strongest, health scientists and health professionals often use evidence hierarchies. An *evidence hierarchy,* or *evidence pyramid,* is typically arranged such that filtered information (synthesized research), or information with the lowest risk for bias, appears at the top, while unfiltered information (single studies) is shown on the bottom. In between, scientific evidence is ordered from strongest to weakest, with slight differences in the numbering of the levels.

To be more specific, although evidence pyramids differ, they are generally organized from top to bottom as follows (see Figure 2.1) (Central Michigan University Libraries, 2018; Dartmouth College, 2006; O'Mathúna & Fineout-Overholt, 2015; Oregon Health & Science University, 2018):

> Individuals may conduct searches for evidence-based sources of information classified as filtered and unfiltered in the Turning Research Into Practice (TRIP) database. This free resource is available at https://www.tripdatabase.com/.

1. Meta-analyses and systematic reviews

2. Critically appraised individual articles (article synopses) and EBP guidelines

3. Randomized controlled trials (RCTs)

4. Non-randomized controlled trials

5. Cohort studies or time series/case series comparisons

6. Case studies or case series

7. Individual case reports, qualitative and descriptive studies, and EBP or quality-improvement (QI) projects

8. Background information or expert opinion

Policy scientists and health professionals who intend to influence the policy discussion must be as meticulous in their search for and use of evidence as clinicians engaged in EBM and EBP. But in policymaking, what constitutes evidence must accommodate the nature of the policymaking process and environment. While the rigidity of standard hierarchies of evidence serves the need to search for scientific evidence to inform policy, additional, more-flexible searching is usually necessary. The definition of evidence, for the purpose of quality policymaking, was established by the UK Cabinet Office (1999) as:

> Expert knowledge; existing domestic and international research; existing statistics; stakeholder consultation; evaluation of previous policies; new research, if appropriate; or secondary sources, including the internet . . . analysis of the outcome of consultation, costings of policy options and the results of economic or statistical modeling. (p. 33)

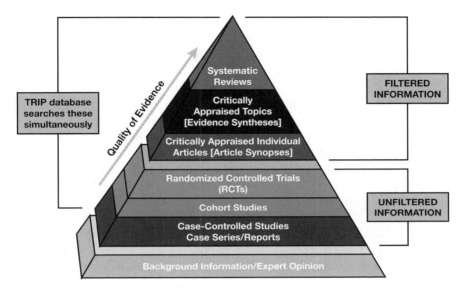

FIGURE 2.1 The EBM pyramid.
(Originally produced by Dartmouth College and Yale University in 2006)

This definition is more inclusive than what is demonstrated by EBM pyramids and reflects the breadth of evidence needed in policymaking. Marston and Watts (2003) noted that, for the purpose of policymaking, there is a "very wide range of what can—properly—count as evidence, based on a premise about the irreducible richness and complexity of social reality" (p. 143).

The same authors made observations about the debate that emerged in the early 2000s about the relative value of a continuum of research and other forms of evidence in policymaking. At one end of the continuum is the rational actor model, which favors the use of research. In contrast, the political model, on the other end of the continuum, views research as one of many contributions to a body of evidence considered during the policymaking process. The authors further explored the fact of this continuum and the power of hierarchies of evidence that prefer a limited range of what constitutes good and appropriate knowledge:

> This comment on the preferred forms of evidence uncovers the potential problems of adopting a narrow view of what counts as valid knowledge . . . If knowledge operates hierarchically, we begin

> to see that far from being a neutral concept, evidence-based policy
> is a powerful metaphor in shaping what forms of knowledge are
> considered closest to the "truth" in decision-making processes and
> policy argument. (p. 145)

In addition to a debate about what evidence is appropriate for use, examples
in the literature caution policymakers about the risks inherent in how evidence
and other source materials are interpreted to reach conclusions that shape
policy. Boaz and Pawson (2005) explain this problem, noting how different
conclusions can be drawn by different teams analyzing the same data. Therefore, the problem "is that fuzzy inferences are then dressed and delivered as
hard evidence [and] deemed to speak for the 'evidence base'" (p. 188).

This discussion grounds the debate about what might constitute the boundaries of evidence to inform evidence-based policymaking. Health scientists
are most familiar with gold-standard forms of scientific evidence, in which
research at the top of the evidence pyramid is held as closest to truth and at
the lowest risk for interpretation bias. But in policymaking, the problems upon
which evidence is called to inform are complicated by the political and complex nature of the policymaking environment. Therefore, problems with using
even the highest levels of evidence may emerge. For example, evidence may be
(Montuschi, 2009):

- **Uncertain:** Examples of this are the long-term impacts of sweeping
  change in healthcare funding.

- **Open to different interpretations:** For example, people interpret the
  effectiveness and risks of certain immunizations in different ways.

- **Misunderstood:** An example of this is the confusion over the effects of
  climate change on respiratory disease in specific regions.

- **Challenged by competing values:** The effect of gun control on the
  safety of schoolchildren is an example of this.

To overcome these limitations, Montuschi (2009) posited the need to raise
three questions central to the discussion of what constitutes evidence:

- **How do certain types of facts candidate themselves as evidence? (p.
  427):** The point of basing policy on reliable evidence is to reduce the
  risk of bias and arbitrary decision-making. General wisdom and the
  evidence hierarchy indicate that empirical evidence is the best way

to do this. Policymaking holds that evidence "for a policy conclusion should make the conclusion probable" (p. 428), so the task is to determine the best kind of evidence to serve this purpose. To that end, the evidence hierarchies used in EBM and EBP may not translate directly because they may not offer the best evidence for use in every context, and because other forms of evidence, typically considered more biased on the evidence hierarchy, might be more effective for reaching a specific policy conclusion.

- **How do we decide what evidence we have, and how much of it? (p. 431):** Relying on scientific evidence is essential, but scientific evidence should be considered judiciously. For example, there are different ways to calculate and present the risks and benefits of a health procedure (such as a screening); relative risk reduction (for example, how screening for certain diseases might reduce the risk of dying by a certain percentage); absolute risk reduction (for example, how screening for certain diseases might reduce the number of persons who die by that disease by percentage points, such as 1 out of 1,000); or number of persons who needed to be screened (for example, to prevent 1 death in a given time frame).

- **Can we combine evidence? (p. 433):** The question Montuschi asks here relates to how relevant evidence from different sources can be combined to acquire levels of objectivity and sufficiency to support a policy decision.

The difficulty in complex and controversial policy issues is in determining whether the conclusion arrived at, based on a body of evidence, is balanced and indicates a reasonable probability of policy success. This is no small task for two reasons, which are addressed here in brief and amplified throughout the text:

- **Absolute objectivity is an ideal that is rarely achieved in policymaking.** The policymaking process is complicated by multiple factors such as partisan politics, political agendas, policymakers' personal interests and agendas, legislative cycles, and many other factors.

- **The ability to apply the policy to real-world government and/or social programs is essential.** Once a policy is enacted, it should be effective at the implementation level, it should serve the citizens it is intended to serve, and it should be reasonable for government or other agencies to implement.

Implications of the Use of Hierarchical Evidence in Policymaking

While established hierarchies of scientific evidence are essential for determining the kinds of evidence required to address clinical practice questions, they may not ideally serve the needs for informing a given health policy. That robust evidence is needed for policymakers to make well-informed decisions is not in question. What constitutes robust evidence to inform a good policy solution is the question that needs to be answered—and the answer depends on the policy question.

There are several implications to consider:

- Expert opinion from reputable sources, which resides at the bottom of classic evidence hierarchies, is generally informed by robust evidence, including methodologically rigorous scientific research.

- Research that is well designed, executed, and reported is more likely to be convincing to policymakers, regardless of its methodological design (for example, descriptive or qualitative studies versus RCTs).

- During the process of gathering and appraising evidence, it is critical to make systematic decisions about what types of evidence are best to inform decision-making for a particular policy. As discussed, context is important in policymaking, and evidence is context-sensitive; therefore, you must make judgments about the applicability of the evidence to the policy problem at hand.

There are challenges inherent in efficiently and effectively using evidence to inform policy decisions. One is the large volume of research evidence available to inform any given problem. Another is how to adapt that evidence to apply at the local policy level. Systematic reviews can be of significant assistance in matters such as these.

Although there are both benefits and disadvantages to using systematic reviews to inform policymaking, and arguments for continuing to enlarge and improve the store of systematic reviews for this purpose have been made (Fox, 2017; Lavis, 2009; Lavis et al., 2005), applying certain strategies can improve the use of systematic reviews in policy decision-making. One is to use summaries of systematic reviews that make the findings more accessible to a broad range of readers, including policymakers; these are called *information products.*

Another is for decision-makers to work directly with specialist groups who can synthesize the evidence in such a way that it is more understandable and therefore more useful during the process (Murthy et al., 2012).

The important takeaway from this discussion is that a broad interpretation of evidence should be understood to include more than research-based evidence (Oliver, Innvar, Lorenc, Woodman, & Thomas, 2014), and that a body of evidence to inform a particular policy may legitimately find excellent sources in the lower tiers of the evidence hierarchy.

> Although policy problems may apply to a local context or population, it is wise to look to global evidence—that is, evidence available from around the world—to avoid limiting evidence collection to a narrow context that could result in an error in judgment. That said, locally relevant evidence, such as disease prevalence, resource availability, economic factors, or anticipated program delivery issues, should also be considered (Oxman et al., 2009).

Sources of Guidance for Evaluating Evidence to Inform Policymaking

A number of sources are available to guide users in evaluating evidence. Three of these are addressed here:

- The World Health Organization (WHO) Grading of Recommendations Assessment Development and Evaluation (GRADE) system
- The Campbell Collaboration
- Results for America

The WHO GRADE System

The WHO GRADE system was developed to rate the quality of evidence and the strength of recommendations in systematic reviews in health technology assessments and clinical practice guidelines (WHO, 2012). The GRADE system provides explicit rating criteria and establishes a logical approach for formulating questions for evaluation and using summary findings tables (Guyatt, Oxman, Kunz, et al., 2011).

A series of articles in the *Journal of Clinical Epidemiology* describes the GRADE system:

- "Framing the Questions and Deciding on Important Outcomes" (Guyatt, Oxman, Kunz, et al., 2011)

- "Rating the Quality of Evidence" (Balshem et al., 2011)

- "Rating the Quality of Evidence-Study Limitations (Risk of Bias)" (Guyatt, Oxman, Vist, et al., 2011)

- "Rating the Quality of Evidence-Publication Bias" (Guyatt, Oxman, Montori, et al., 2011)

After publishing the GRADE guidelines, the WHO published the *WHO Handbook for Guideline Development* (2012) to assist with the development of clinical, public health, and policy guidelines. The GRADE guidelines are embedded in this handbook and continue to serve as the foundation for the current standard. Updates have addressed best practices to improve GRADE evidence tables and the grading of evidence (Carrasco-Labra et al., 2016; Langendam et al., 2016; Santesso et al., 2016).

The Campbell Collaboration

A more accessible and user-friendly source of information for the layperson, stakeholder, policymaker, or health professional is the Campbell Collaboration. The Campbell Collaboration, based in Oslo, Norway, states that its mission is to promote "positive social and economic change through the production and use of systematic reviews and other evidence synthesis for evidence based policy and practice" (2018). Its Better Evidence page includes links to systematic reviews, plain language summaries (summaries of its systematic reviews), and policy briefs (brief summaries of its systematic reviews). Major categories, called *coordinating groups,* include titles that are directly or indirectly related to health policy issues—for example, nutrition or social welfare.

Results for America

A third organization that provides useful information and guidance on evidence for use in policymaking is Results for America. Its mission:

> . . . is helping decision-makers at all levels of government harness the power of evidence and data to solve our world's greatest challenges. Our mission is to make investing in what works the "new normal," so that when policymakers make decisions, they start by seeking the best evidence and data available, then use what they find to get better results. (2018)

Results for America focuses on policymaking in the broad sense rather than health policy specifically. However, it is a useful resource for individuals interested in advancing health policy, as some of its support materials relate directly to health policy issues.

For example, one policy report on evidence-based innovation programs (2015) summarizes the strategic congressional funding of innovation programs that surfaced during the Obama administration. Among these were programs in the Teen Pregnancy Prevention Program (administered by the US Department of Health and Human Services [HHS] Office of Adolescent Health) and in the Maternal, Infant, and Early Childhood Home Visiting Program (administered by the Health Resources and Services Administration at HHS).

Another useful policy report is a brief titled "9 Ways to Make Federal Legislation Evidence-Based: 2017 What Works Guide for Congress," which outlines nine ways that Congress can ensure that the laws they pass are based on evidence. The organization acknowledges that all nine recommendations may not be relevant to all bills but suggests that Congress adhere to those recommendations that are relevant. The recommendations are as follows (Results for America, 2017):

- **Evaluate the effectiveness of federal programs and practices:** This should be accomplished by ensuring that a percentage of program funds will be preserved for agencies to evaluate programs and practices.
- **Define what evidence-based means:** A rigorous, tiered definition of "evidence-based" should be used to ensure federal funds are appropriately invested in solutions with a strong evidence base.

- **Apply the definition of evidence-based to how federal grant funds are allocated:** This means giving funding priority to activities based on the strongest evidence.

- **Authorize a tiered evidence-innovation fund:** This proposes the authorization of a tiered grant program based on the strength of evidence.

- **Provide Pay for Success authority:** This suggests a new form of grant program funding policy that would pay grantees only after delivery of specified results.

- **Increase flexibility for federal grantees in exchange for using data and evidence to improve results:** Enactment of this recommendation would authorize federal agencies to waive federal grant recipient program requirements and allow recipients to implement innovative evidence-based interventions. In exchange, the grantee would be required to rigorously evaluate the new approach.

- **Support appropriate sharing and use of data and evidence:** This involves instituting a publicly available and easily used clearinghouse to disseminate evidence-based interventions.

- **Repurpose federal funds away from practices, grantees, and programs that consistently fail to achieve desired outcomes:** This means using evaluations and outcomes data to eliminate low-performing federal grantees, requiring them to re-apply and compete with other grant-seekers to continue federal funding.

- **Use federal funds to build state and local capacity:** This recommendation requires federal agencies to provide technical and other assistance to federal grantees at all levels as they build and use evidence.

Examples of the Use and Influence of Evidence on Policymaking and Practice

Now that you are aware of the various kinds of evidence, the question becomes, how effective are these kinds of evidence in health policymaking? The answer is, it depends on the policy problem. This section contains two examples that illustrate this assertion. The first example discusses a much-needed change in state law to permit expedited partner therapy (EPT) and demonstrates how a variety of sources, from different levels of the evidence hierarchy, were used to craft public policy. The second example illustrates variations in mammography screening guidelines across several organizations based on differences in evidence interpretation. (Mammography screening guidelines do not have the force and effect of law, but they are influential in that they guide practice and influence third-party payers.) How the organizations and agencies in these examples used established evidence hierarchies may have been similar, but how evidence was interpreted and used to inform their guidelines (which are, in effect, policy) differed.

Example 1: A State Law Permitting EPT

A few years ago, Ohio was one of the last four states that still prohibited EPT. As explained by the Centers for Disease Control and Prevention (CDC), EPT is "the clinical practice of treating the sex partners of patients diagnosed with chlamydia or gonorrhea by providing prescriptions or medications to the patient to take to his/her partner without the healthcare provider first examining the partner" (CDC, 2017).

Legislators used several categories of evidence to inform their decision to update state law. A key evidence source was the CDC's "Review and Guidance" document, published in 2006. Although it did not meet the standard five-year rule for currency in healthcare science, it was the most recent CDC document on that topic, and no new evidence had emerged. Indeed, the document remains the gold standard for guiding EPT practice. It includes a review of clinical practice, a systematic review of the evidence that incorporates results of relevant RCTs and other types of rigorous research, and recommendations for implementing EPT in practice (CDC, 2006). This document constitutes what is known as an *evidence-based clinical guideline* and is classified as expert opinion, generally relegated to the lowest level on the evidence hierarchy. However, as mentioned, it contains an embedded systematic review of the literature, which includes RCTs and other forms of rigorous research.

Lawmakers also accessed state health department data reports on the incidence of the three most common and treatable STIs included in the EPT cluster (including *C. trachomatis*). This is considered internal (state-specific) data, otherwise known as "local" evidence. Additionally, they explored the literature on re-infection rates if sexually transmitted infections are left untreated, co-morbidities such as pelvic inflammatory disease and infertility, and studies and reports from other states that had implemented EPT laws. It is impossible to discern, from the policymakers' point of view, whether they prioritized their consideration of the evidence (that is, they gave more weight to evidence higher on the evidence pyramid), or whether the body of evidence described constituted a full dossier of information, with each piece given equal weight in informing their discussion and facilitating their decision-making. Regardless, the evidence was effective in leveraging both dialogue and conservative partisan politics, and the bill passed.

Example 2: Differing Recommendations for Mammography Screening

Four reputable, US-based national organizations, including the US Preventive Services Task Force, have published related but somewhat conflicting recommendations for breast cancer screening for women of average risk, all based on interpretations of the best available evidence. It is irrefutable that screening mammography reduces breast cancer mortality rates in women aged 39 to 69 (Nelson et al., 2009). However, the age at which it should begin and whether clinical adjuncts such as breast self-exam or clinical examination should be offered are less clear.

Table 2.1 notes the four organizations and summarizes areas of guideline agreement and disagreement. (Three additional organizations that publish breast cancer screening guidelines are not included. These are the American College of Radiology, which focuses on high-risk women; the National Comprehensive Cancer Network, omitted because it is a private nonprofit organization rather than profession- or government-based; and the Canadian Task Force on Preventive Health Care, omitted because it is not based in the US. However, a thorough examination and comparison could include all seven of these organizations.)

TABLE 2.1: A Comparison of Mammography Screening Guidelines for Women of Average Risk

Screening Method	American Academy of Family Physicians (2013)*	American Cancer Society (2015)**	American College of Obstetricians and Gynecologists (2017)***	US Preventive Services Task Force (2016)****
Breast self-examination	Recommends against (no reduction in mortality)	Does not recommend (qualified)	Does not recommend (qualified: self-awareness aids detection)	Does not recommend
Clinical breast examination	Evidence insufficient (an option but does not replace screening mammography)	Does not recommend (qualified)	May offer every 1-3 years for women age 25-39; annually for women 40 years and older	Insufficient evidence
Mammography	Recommends routine biennial screening for women age 50-74	Recommends routine annual screening for women age 45-54. Recommends biennial screening for women age 55 and older; option to continue annually; stop when life expectancy less than 10 years	Recommends annual or biennial screening for women age 40-49 after counseling if patient desires. Recommends screening by no later than age 50 and continuing until age 75	Recommends biennial screening for women age 50-74. For women age 40-49 years, recommends individual decision based on risk versus benefit analysis. For women 75 and older, does not recommend (evidence insufficient)

*Tirona, 2013

**Oeffinger et al., 2015

***American College of Obstetricians and Gynecologists, 2017

****US Preventive Services Task Force, 2016

Interestingly, each of these organizations interpreted and applied a legitimate body of evidence in a responsible manner to support its policy decisions. Moreover, each organization seeks to protect patients, mitigate potential risks of false positives, and guide clinicians. And yet, each came to different conclusions. This case exemplifies Oxman and colleagues' (2009) view that "evidence can be used to support a conclusion, but it is not the same as a conclusion. *Evidence alone does not make decisions . . .* " (p. 3) (emphasis added).

The Changing Perspectives on the Use of Evidence and Big Data

Any conversation about the broad range of evidence used in policymaking must include a discussion about the use of big data and its implications. Hebda (2019) defines *big data* as "very large data sets beyond human capability to analyze or manage without the aid of technology used to reveal patterns and discover new learning" (p. 133).

Healthcare data sets, nontraditional data streams from internet-based platforms and applications, electronic health records, and other sources of big data are becoming increasingly available and have great potential for use in policymaking. Three areas in which the value of big data may likely be realized include (Hebda, 2019):

- Outcomes from advances in personalized medicine
- The customization of diagnostics, treatment decisions, and patient education to improve health practices and population health analysis
- Support for tools needed for the detection and prevention of healthcare fraud

Advances in technology and analytic capabilities have made the use of big data appealing and potentially beneficial. However, the use of big data is not without its challenges; data security, technology management, and accountability are concerns of paramount importance (Vayena, Dzenowagis, Brownstein, & Sheikh, 2017).

During the Obama administration, the Evidence-Based Policymaking Commission Act of 2016 established the Commission on Evidence-Based Policymaking (CEP). The bill was cosponsored by Speaker of the House Paul Ryan (R-WI) and Senator Patty Murray (D-WA). The purpose of the law was to establish the CEP to develop strategies for increasing the availability and use of data to build evidence to inform government programs and to protect data privacy and confidentiality (CEP, 2017). The CEP released its final report on September 7, 2017, and subsequently reported its recommendations to the full House Committee on Oversight and Government Reform on September 26, 2017 (Committee on Oversight and Government Reform, n.d.).

Recommendations of the CEP encompass four major areas (CEP, 2017):

- Improving secure, private, and confidential data access
- Modernizing privacy protections for evidence building
- Implementing a National Secure Data Service
- Strengthening federal evidence-building capacity

Following the report to the House committee, the US Congress introduced companion bills for translating the four major CEP recommendations into federal policy. One of these was the Foundations for Evidence-Based Policymaking Act of 2017 (Congress.gov, 2017a), introduced in the Senate by Senator Patty Murray on October 31, 2017. The same day, Speaker Paul Ryan introduced a bill by the same title in the House (Congress.gov, 2017b). Murray's bill stalled, but Ryan's was quickly considered by the House Committee on Oversight and Government Reform and passed by the House on November 15, 2017. In the final hours of the 115th Congressional Session, it was passed by the Senate. It was subsequently signed by President Trump on January 14, 2018, and became Public Law No: 115-435.

The CEP clarified the issues surrounding the use of big data with regard to security, privacy, access, and technology. The recommendations are clear, and data privacy watchdog organizations, such as the Electronic Privacy Information Center (EPIC), have come out in support of the recommendations (EPIC, 2017). It is fortunate that a federal bill based on the recommendations has been signed into law, which should serve to mitigate the risks associated with the use of big data as a source of evidence in policymaking.

Strategies for Using Evidence in Policymaking for Nurses and Other Healthcare Professionals

Nurses and other healthcare professionals who are involved in advancing health policy should be aware of the types of legitimate evidence that can be useful in policymaking and search for evidence that will support the most convincing arguments. Experts in public administration have long known that "scientific evidence plays a part in this process, but we should not exaggerate the ability of scientists to win the day with reference to evidence" (Cairney & Oliver, 2016, p. 400). Therefore, gaining wisdom in how to use evidence effectively is essential.

As discussed, evidence from top-pyramid research may be most convincing to research scientists, but it may be less important to the policymakers who must also consider stakeholders, constituents, political relationships, budget cycles, and legislative priorities. For this reason, using a pragmatic approach will likely yield a higher rate of success. Strategies may include packaging evidence to ensure that the science is more accessible and understandable for policymakers, using stories to raise emotion around an issue and exemplify research findings, and framing evidence to demonstrate how its use in policy is realistic (Cairney & Oliver, 2016; Cairney & Oliver, 2017).

One quandary for scientists—and, by extension, health professionals—is that they must determine how to balance the preparation of a body of valid evidence with an emotional and political appeal in such a way that it will deliver an unambiguous and persuasive message to policymakers. Another dilemma is whether the body of evidence should be presented to policymakers in a way that is prioritized more highly than political factors (Cairney & Oliver, 2017). Cairney and Oliver (2017) assert that these decisions are value-driven and political rather than driven by evidence. The best decision is arrived at by weighing the political environment and policy actors against the body of evidence as it stands.

Considering the changing landscape of evidence in the current policymaking environment, the following suggestions may be of use:

- Keep expectations of the use of evidence realistic. Evidence is used to inform dialogue and decision-making, not as an absolute policy driver. Policymakers must balance evidence with a multitude of other political factors.

- When searching for evidence, the best evidence to inform policy might *not* be found at the top of the evidence pyramid. Make judgments about what constitutes legitimate evidence to inform a particular policy.

- Make certain the body of evidence disseminated to policymakers is accurately interpreted and described. Avoid interpreting literature to stack the deck in favor of your policy.

- Package the body of evidence to make it accessible to the lay public and policymakers.

- Use big data if it is useful for addressing a particular policy problem.

Summary

This chapter explored the emerging and controversial uses of science, research, and evidence in policymaking and what constitutes legitimate evidence in this milieu. In the health sciences, research that resides closer to the top of the evidence pyramid or hierarchy is considered the most rigorous and therefore the best. This is not always the case in policymaking, however. Methodologically sound research at other levels of the hierarchy, including expert opinion and evidence-based guidelines, can provide a wealth of useful evidence.

This chapter also provided a non-exhaustive overview of sources of information on the use of evidence in policymaking, including the WHO GRADE system, the Campbell Collaboration, and Results for America. Examples of the use of evidence and its influence on public health policy and practice were provided, including a stunning example of variations in evidence interpretation in the issuing of recommendations for mammography screening for women of average risk.

Changing perspectives on the use of evidence and of big data were also addressed. The issue of privacy with respect to the use of big data in particular has recently come to the attention of policymakers thanks to recommendations issued by the CEP, resulting in the introduction of companion bills in the US Congress.

Finally, the chapter addressed how to make the best use of evidence in policymaking and offered strategies for nurses and other healthcare professionals.

References

American College of Obstetricians and Gynecologists, Committee on Practice Bulletins—Gynecology. (2017). Breast cancer risk assessment and screening in average-risk women. *ACOG Practice Bulletin,* Number 179. Retrieved from https://www.acog.org/-/media/Practice-Bulletins/Committee-on-Practice-Bulletins----Gynecology/Public/pb179.pdf?dmc=1&ts=20181214T1806345987

Balshem, H., Helfand, M., Schünemann, H. J., Oxman, A. D., Kunz, R., Brozek, J., . . . Guyatt, G. H. (2011). GRADE guidelines: 3. Rating the quality of evidence. *Journal of Clinical Epidemiology, 64*(4), 401–406. doi:10.1016/j.clinepi.2010.07.015

Boaz, A., & Pawson, R. (2005). The perilous road from evidence to policy: Five journeys compared. *Journal of Social Policy, 34*(2), 175–194. doi:10.1017/S0047279404008530

Cairney, P., & Oliver, K. (2016). To bridge the divide between evidence and policy: Reduce ambiguity as much as uncertainty. *Public Administration Review, 76*(3), 399–402. doi:10.1111/puar.12555

Cairney, P., & Oliver, K. (2017). Evidence-based policymaking is not like evidence-based medicine, so how far should you go to bridge the divide between evidence and policy? *Health Research Policy and Systems, 15*(35). doi:10.1186/s12961-017-0192-x

Campbell Collaboration. (2018). Better evidence. Retrieved from https://campbellcollaboration.org/better-evidence.html

Carrasco-Labra, A., Brignardello-Petersen, R., Santesso, N., Neumann, I., Mustafa, R. A., Mbuagbaw, L., . . . Schünemann, H. J. (2016). Improving GRADE evidence tables part 1: A randomized trial shows improved understanding of content in summary of findings tables with a new format. *Journal of Clinical Epidemiology, 74*, 7–18. doi:10.1016.j.clinepi.2015.12.007

Centers for Disease Control and Prevention. (2006). *Expedited partner therapy in the management of sexually transmitted diseases.* Retrieved from https://www.cdc.gov/std/treatment/eptfinalreport2006.pdf

Centers for Disease Control and Prevention. (2017). Expedited partner therapy. Retrieved from https://www.cdc.gov/std/ept/default.htm

Central Michigan University Libraries. (2018). Evidence-based medicine: Resources by levels of evidence. Retrieved from https://libguides.cmich.edu/cmed/ebm/pyramid

Commission on Evidence-Based Policymaking. (2017). *The promise of evidence-based policymaking.* Retrieved from https://www.cep.gov/content/dam/cep/report/cep-final-report.pdf

Committee on Oversight and Government Reform. (n.d.). Recommendations of the Commission on Evidence-Based Policymaking. Retrieved from https://oversight.house.gov/hearing/recommendations-commission-evidence-based-policymaking/

Congress.gov. (2017a). S.2046–Foundations for Evidence-Based Policymaking Act of 2017. Retrieved from https://www.congress.gov/bill/115th-congress/senate-bill/2046

Congress.gov. (2017b). H.R.4174–Foundations for Evidence-Based Policymaking Act of 2017. Retrieved from https://www.congress.gov/bill/115th-congress/house-bill/4174/actions

Dartmouth College. (2006). Evidence-based mental health resources. Retrieved from http://www.dartmouth.edu/~biomed/resources.htmld/guides/ebm_psych_resources.html

Electronic Privacy Information Center. (2017). EPIC backs Commission on Evidence-Based Policymaking, urges Congress to take steps to preserve privacy. Retrieved from https://epic.org/2017/09/epic-praises-recommendations-o.html

Fox, D. M. (2017). Evidence and health policy: Using and regulating systematic reviews. *American Journal of Public Health, 107*(1), 88–92.

Guyatt, G. H., Oxman, A. D., Kunz, R., Atkins, D., Brozek, J., Vist, G., . . . Schünemann, H. J. (2011). GRADE guidelines: 2. Framing the question and deciding on important outcomes. *Journal of Clinical Epidemiology, 64*(4), 395–400. doi:10.1016/jclinepi.2010.09.012

Guyatt, G. H., Oxman, A. D., Montori, V., Vist, G., Kunz, R., Brozek, J., . . . Schünemann, H. J. (2011). GRADE guidelines: 5. Rating the quality of evidence–publication bias. *Journal of Clinical Epidemiology, 64*(12), 1277–1282. doi:10.1016/j.jclinepi.2011.01.011

Guyatt, G. H., Oxman, A. D., Vist, G., Kunz, R., Brozek, J., Alonso-Coello, P., . . . Schünemann, H. J. (2011). GRADE guidelines: 4. Rating the quality of evidence-study limitations (risk of bias). *Journal of Clinical Epidemiology, 64*(4), 407–415. doi:10.1016/j.jclinepi.2010.07.017

Hall, J. L., & Jennings, E. T. (2010). Assessing the use and weight of information and evidence in U.S. state policy decisions. *Policy and Society, 29*(2), 137–147.

Hebda, T. (2019). The impact of EHRs, big data, and evidence-informed practice. In J. A. Milstead & N. M. Short (Eds.), *Health policy and politics: A nurse's guide* (pp. 133–150). Burlington, MA: Jones & Bartlett Learning.

Langendam, M., Carrasco-Labra, A., Santesso, N., Mustafa, R. A., Brignardello-Peterson, R., Ventresca, M., . . . Schünemann, H. J. (2016). Improving GRADE evidence tables part 2: A systematic survey of explanatory notes shows more guidance is needed. *Journal of Clinical Epidemiology, 74,* 19–27. doi:10.1016/j.jclinepi.2015.12.008

Lavis, J. N. (2009). How can we support the use of systematic reviews in policymaking? *PLoS Medicine, 6*(11), e1000141. Retrieved from http://journals.plos.org/plosmedicine/article/file?id=10.1371/journal.pmed.1000141&type=printable

Lavis, J., Davies, H., Oxman, A., Denis, J. L., Golden-Biddle, K., & Ferlie, E. (2005). Towards systematic reviews that inform health care management and policy-making. *Journal of Health Services Research and Policy, 10*(Suppl. 1), 35–48.

Lomas, J., Culyer, T., McCutcheon, C., McAuley, L., & Law, S. (2005) *Conceptualizing and combining evidence for health system guidance.* Canadian Health Services Research Foundation. Retrieved from https://www.cfhi-fcass.ca/migrated/pdf/insightAction/evidence_e.pdf

Marston, G., & Watts, R. (2003) Tampering with the evidence: A critical appraisal of evidence-based policy-making. *The Drawing Board: An Australian Review of Public Affairs, 3*(3), 143–163.

Maynard, R. A. (2006). Evidence-based decision making: What will it take for the decision makers to care? *Journal of Policy Analysis and Management, 25*(2), 249–265.

Montuschi, E. (2009). Questions of evidence in evidence-based policy. *Axiomathes, 19,* 425–439. doi:10.1007/s10516-009-9085-0

Murthy, L., Shepperd, S., Clarke, M. J., Garner, S. E., Lavis, J. N., Perrier, L., . . . Straus, S. E. (2012). Interventions to improve the use of systematic reviews in decision-making by health system managers, policy makers and clinicians. *Cochrane Database of Systematic Reviews,* Issue 9, CD009401. doi:10.1002/14651858.CD009401.pub2

Nelson, H. D., Tyne, K., Naik, A., Bougatsos, C., Chan, B. K., & Humphrey, L. (2009) Screening for breast cancer: An update for the U.S. Preventive Services Task Force. *Annals of Internal Medicine, 151*(10), 727–737. doi:10.7326/0003-4819-151-10-200911170-00009

Oeffinger, K. C., Fontham, E. T. H., Etzioni, R., Herzig, A., Michaelson, J. S., Shih, Y. T., ... Wender, R. (2015). Breast cancer screening for women at average risk: 2015 guideline update from the American Cancer Society. *Journal of the American Medical Association, 314*(15), 1599–1614. doi:10.1001/jama.2015.12783

Oliver, K., Innvar, S., Lorenc, T., Woodman, J., & Thomas, J. (2014). A systematic review of barriers to and facilitators of the use of evidence by policymakers. *BMC Health Services Research, 14*(2). doi:10.1186/1472-6963-14-2

O'Mathúna, D. P., & Fineout-Overholt, E. (2015). Critically appraising quantitative evidence for clinical decision making. In B. M. Melnyk & E. Fineout-Overholt (Eds.), *Evidence-based practice in nursing & healthcare: A guide to best practice* (3rd ed., pp. 87–138). Philadelphia, PA: Lippincott Williams & Wilkins.

Oregon Health & Science University. (2018). Johns Hopkins Nursing EBP: Levels of evidence. Retrieved from http://libguides.ohsu.edu/ebptoolkit/levelsofevidence

Oxman, A. D., Lavis, J. N., Lewin, S., & Fretheim, A. (2009). SUPPORT tools for evidence-informed health policymaking (STP) 1: What is evidence-informed policymaking? *Health Research Policy and Systems, 7*(Suppl. 1). doi:10.1186/1478- 4505-7-S1-S1

Results for America. (2015). Invest in what works fact sheet: Evidence-based innovation programs. Retrieved from https://results4america.org/tools/invest-works-fact-sheet-federal-evidence-based-innovation-programs/

Results for America. (2017). 9 ways to make federal legislation evidence-based: 2017 what works guide for Congress. Retrieved from https://results4america.org/tools/works-legislation-9-ways-make-federal-legislation-evidence-based/

Results for America. (2018). Our mission. Retrieved from https://results4america.org/about-us/

Santesso, N., Carrasco-Labra, A., Langendam, M., Brignardello-Peterson, R., Mustafa, R.A., Heus, P., . . . Schünemann, H. J. (2016). Improving GRADE evidence tables part 3: Detailed guidance for explanatory footnotes supports creating and understanding GRADE certainty in the evidence judgments. *Journal of Clinical Epidemiology, 74*, 28–39. doi:10.1016/j.jclinepi.2015.12.006

Tirona, M. T. (2013). Breast cancer screening update. *American Family Physician, 87*(4), 274–278.

UK Cabinet Office. (1999). *Professional policy making for the twenty first century*. Retrieved from http://dera.ioe.ac.uk/6320/1/profpolicymaking.pdf

US Preventive Services Task Force. (2016). *Final recommendation statement: Breast cancer screening*. Retrieved from https://www.uspreventiveservicestaskforce.org/Page/Document/RecommendationStatementFinal/breast-cancer-screening1

Vayena, E., Dzenowagis, J., Brownstein, J. S., & Sheikh, A. (2017). Policy implications of big data in the health sector. *Bulletin of the World Health Organization, 96*, 66–68. doi:10.2471/BLT.17.197426

World Health Organization. (2012). *WHO handbook for guideline development*. Retrieved from http://apps.who.int/iris/bitstream/handle/10665/75146/9789241548441_eng.pdf; jsessionid=5C54D7963C8FD221E83ACEA45E9B7C8D?sequence=1

"Consistently wise decisions can only be made by those whose wisdom is constantly challenged."

–Theodore C. Sorensen

3

HEALTH POLICY AND POLITICS

–JOYCE ZURMEHLY, PHD, DNP, RN, NEA-BC, ANEF

KEY CONTENT IN THIS CHAPTER

- Key terms related to health policy
- Health policy as an entity and as a process
- Differentiating the big P and little p in health policy
- Politics in health policymaking
- Nurses and health policy
- Chaos theory, the butterfly effect, and the charge to advance health policy change

Key Terms Related to Health Policy

The influence of health policy on healthcare in the United States has been of concern to the public since President Truman's administration. Healthcare reform and efforts to advance health policy (or stall progress) have been highlighted during every congressional session since that time.

Fueled by media coverage and partisan politics, public concern over issues related to health and the policies that address those issues continues to grow. Public anxiety escalates due to concern over incidents such as the measles outbreak connected to Disneyland in California and subsequent calls for mandatory childhood vaccines, and the Ebola outbreak in the western African countries of Guinea, Sierra Leone, and Liberia and potential pandemic thereafter (Apollonio & Bero, 2016). The long-term future of the Patient Protection and Affordable Care Act (ACA) is also a cause for concern. After an initial substantial increase in people covered in the individual insurance market (up 64% to 17.4 million people) in 2015, enrollments remained relatively unchanged in 2016. However, they declined after that in response to disagreements about the act's future in Congress and an uncertain third-party payer market—although 14.4 million people remain enrolled (Semanskee, Levitt, & Cox, 2018).

Whether they involve a healthcare concern or health reform, these examples show how individual attitudes and public concerns shape health policy and help set the stage for discussions on what exactly constitutes health policy. To aid readers in that discussion, this section defines and explores several key terms: policy, public policy, and health policy.

Policy

According to Black, a *policy* is understood to be:

> the general principles by which a government is guided in its management of public affairs, or the legislature in its measure. This term, as applied to a law, ordinance, or rule of law, denotes its general purpose or tendency considered as directed to the policy. (n.d.-a)

Policy refers to decisions made by an authority about an action—either one to be taken or one to be prohibited—to promote or limit the occurrence of a particular circumstance in a population. In the public sector, the authority charged with making health policy is a legislative, executive, or judicial body operating under the authority of a federal, state, or local public administration. In summary, policy describes the general principles a government uses to manage its public affairs.

Public Policy

Public policy is more specific, in that it includes, according to Black:

> the policies that have been declared by the state that covers the state's citizens. These laws and policies allow the government to stop any action that is against the public's interest. (n.d.-c)

In this definition, the term *state* is used in its broad sense, which is "a body politic, or society [of people] united together for the purpose of promoting their mutual safety and advantage, by the joint efforts of their combined strength" (Black, n.d.-d). Public policy refers to the process of decision-making or to the decisions in fact that have an impact on the general population or on significant segments of the general population. Public policy is meant to improve the conditions and general welfare of the population or subpopulations under its jurisdiction.

Although public policies are intended to serve the interests of the public at large, the term *public* has different interpretations according to the political context in which it is applied. Public policy is the expression, by action or inaction, of governmental will. A broader definition of public policy is that it embraces "government policies that affect the whole population" (Public policy, n.d.). Easton's classic definition of public policy describes "the authoritative allocation of values for the whole society" and is one of the few definitions that is straightforward in describing the commanding, if somewhat imposing, role of policymakers in the public process (1953, p. 129).

Only the government can act authoritatively for the whole society. In accordance with this point of view, what government chooses to do (or not to do) results in the "allocation of values." Public policies are in effect authoritative decisions made by the legislative, executive, or judicial branches of government, by individuals serving in their official elected or appointed roles and capacities. These decisions are intended to direct or influence the actions, behaviors, or decisions of others (Longest, 1998).

Health Policy

Health policy is:

> the development by government and other policy makers of present and future objectives pertaining to health care and the health care system, and the articulation of arguments and decisions regarding these objectives in legislation, judicial opinions, regulations, guidelines, standards, etc. that affect health care and public health. (US National Library of Medicine, 2004)

When public policies or authoritative decisions pertain to health or influence the pursuit of healthcare, they become health policies (Hlavac, Beagley, & Zucchi, 2018). Forms of health policy include the following:

- Decisions made by legislators that are subsequently codified in enacted legislation
- Rules or regulations that amplify statutory law and are promulgated (written or established) by executive branch regulatory agencies to implement legislation or operate government programs
- Judicial decisions related to law or regulation

Examples of health policies include the following (Longest, 1998):

- The 1965 federal law establishing the Medicare and Medicaid programs
- An executive order regarding the operation of federally funded health centers
- A court ruling indicating that an integrated delivery system's acquisition of another hospital violates federal antitrust laws
- A state law for licensing a category of healthcare professionals

A more global definition of health policy notes that it "refers to decisions, plans, and actions that are undertaken to achieve specific health care goals within a society" (World Health Organization [WHO], 2018).

Health policy should be distinguished from *healthcare policy* (Shi, 2013), which refers to that part of health policy pertaining to the financing, organization, and delivery of care. Healthcare policy might cover the following:

- The training of health professionals
- The licensing of health professionals and facilities
- The administration of public health insurance programs, such as Medicare and Medicaid
- The deployment of electronic health records
- Efforts to control healthcare costs
- The regulation of private health insurance

The primary goal of health policy is to improve population health, whereas the goals of healthcare policy are typically to provide equitable and efficient access to, and quality of, needed healthcare services.

The Relationship Between Policy and the Health of Populations

Health policy can be broadly defined as policy that pertains to or influences the "development by government and other policy makers of . . . objectives pertaining to [the] attainment of health" (US National Library of Medicine, 2004), and the "decisions, plans and actions undertaken to achieve specific health care goals within a society" (WHO, 2018). In terms of the determinants-of-health framework, health policy refers to legislation as well as other forms of policy such as judicial opinions, regulations, guidelines, or standards that may directly or indirectly influence social and physical environments, behaviors, socioeconomic status, and availability of and accessibility to medical care services (Shi, 2013).

Health policies affect groups or classes of individuals, such as physicians, nurses, pharmacists, and other healthcare providers, as well as citizen and population groups, including the underserved, the elderly, and children. Health policies can also affect types of organizations, such as medical schools, HMOs, nursing homes, medical technology producers, and employers. Health consequences may result directly or indirectly from virtually all major health policies and affect a variety of citizen groups; such policies include but are not limited to Social Security mandates, national defense–related guidelines, labor policy, and immigration policy (Shi, 2013). When special interest and watchdog groups, and our congressional representatives, understand the potential relationship between the health of populations and many of the policies that are established by government—whether they are directly related to health programs or not— the health of populations, particularly vulnerable populations, is better served.

Health Policy as an Entity and as a Process

Health policy can be defined as the development of objectives that pertain to both healthcare and healthcare systems by government and other policy makers. These objectives may be established in arguments and decisions that are actualized in products. The products include legislation, judicial opinions, regulations, guidelines, standards, and others. This definition of health policy includes both verbs (developing) and nouns (objectives and products). There- fore, health policy can be thought of as both an entity and a process.

Health Policy as an Entity

As an entity, health policy includes the standing body of decisions made by those in authority that reflect their views and ideas and provide direction based on their philosophy and mission to those who will carry out the policy. Health policy is made and carried out at all levels of government as well as by the private sector. When health policy is instituted at the governmental level, it has the force and effect of law; when instituted at the organizational level, as in the private sector, it has authority insofar as the organization has authority.

The most commonly referred to policy that constitutes an entity is a law. The term *law* has synonyms, including statute and code. In some states, the state law is referred to as the state's *revised code* (*revised* because it has been changed since its inception). Laws serve as legal directives of behavior for the public. Laws are made by the legislative branch of a government, at the inter- national, federal, state, and local or municipal levels, and are key measures for guiding conduct. Laws are enforceable, with the executive branch of govern- ment serving as the enforcer.

Regulations constitute another type of policy entity. Synonyms for regulation include rule and administrative code. Regulations are written, or promulgated, by the executive branch of a government. For an executive branch agency to have the legal authority to promulgate regulations, the legislation that created that agency must include language that gives the agency explicit rule-making authority. This is called *statutory authority*. Regulations amplify or flesh out law and have the force and effect of law. Examples of regulations specific to health policy include rules written by departments of health and health professions boards—for example, boards of nursing, pharmacy, and medicine.

Other types of policy entities include executive orders, judicial decrees, resolutions, and more. All these entities are formal, tangible outcomes of the policy process.

Health Policy as a Process

Health policy is the process that takes place between the public's dawning awareness of a health issue or problem that might be solved through policy and the enactment of a policy that will address that issue. This process includes the following steps:

1. Setting an agenda

2. Identifying the problem to clarify and frame the issue

3. Performing policy analysis to determine options to address the problem

4. Developing strategy

5. Developing the policy

Policy development includes the process of writing legislation or regulation and following procedures to enact the law or promulgate the regulation (Centers for Disease Control and Prevention [CDC], 2015; Pacheco & Boushey, 2014). The processes of policy implementation and evaluation are also included, following enactment or promulgation (Pacheco & Boushey, 2014).

The health policymaking process is continuous. It is not sequential or necessarily logical. Existing health policies are frequently reviewed to ensure continued relevance and viability of goals and methods (Pacheco & Boushey, 2014). No health policy will ever be adequate to serve the needs of the public indefinitely. Health policies will always require monitoring and adjustment. For this reason, a legal standard known as a *sunset law,* also called a sunset *provision,* has existed in the US since the 1970s and has been promoted as a measure to ensure government efficiency. Sunset laws assist in eliminating government bureaucracies that have become unresponsive or distended by requiring an automatic review and termination on a preset date in statute. The government program, agency, or law is reviewed by the legislature and is terminated unless the legislature affirms renewal in law (Latham, 2018). In this way, sunset provisions force process; they require a review for efficacy, sustainability, and relevancy. The forcing of process ahead of expiration is effective because it is easier and more effective to revise existing law than to allow a law to expire, which would require a lengthy re-introduction and re-legislation process.

Differentiating the Big P and Little P in Health Policy

The colloquial terms for governmental policy versus organizational or private sector policy are *big P* and *little p,* respectively.

Governmental Policy (Big P)

Government policy is known as big policy, or big P. Health policy problems that require a government response and solution must occur on the governmental stage. Regardless of whether that governmental stage is at the macro level (global, federal, or state) or micro level (local or municipal), big P refers to a policy entity that has the force and effect of law. Therefore, big Ps must be established through public policy processes. All the policy entities discussed earlier that have the force and effect of law qualify, such as law, regulation, taxes, and public budgets. Presidential executive orders, judicial decrees, attorney general opinions, and other policies that are produced by government structures also constitute big Ps.

Organizational Policy (Little P)

By contrast, little policy, or little p, refers to those entity policies that are executed by a nongovernmental organization. These policies have a force and effect of a different scale. They may have an effect on a small scale, as with policies made for implementation within a workplace. Or, they may have an effect on a global scale—for example, if the little p is a position statement that offers an evidence-based guideline related to the care of people with a certain communicable disease.

In healthcare institutions, policies and procedures for patient care—which should emerge from evidence-based guidelines or another evidence base— become little p for that organization. Additional examples of organization-specific policies include policies pertaining to staff recruitment, conflict resolution, employee codes of conduct, internal and external relationships, confidentiality, compensation, safety and security, and ethics. Others may include policies pertaining to employee relations and benefits; organizational and employee development; information, communication, and technology issues; and corporate social-involvement policies.

Unlike governmental policy, organizational policy at the private-sector level serves as an important form of internal control. Individuals typically partici-pate in policymaking at the organizational level to influence the allocation of resources or implement change.

Little p is also produced by larger organizations and associations—for ex-ample, professional associations, recognition and accreditation organizations, and nongovernmental organizations (NGOs). The Joint Commission produces policy that qualifies as little p. Its standards are not law, but organizations ac-credited by The Joint Commission must abide by those standards or jeopardize losing that accreditation. Consequences of the loss of accreditation are severe in terms of federal reimbursement and organizational reputation. Eligibility requirements for the ANCC Magnet Recognition Program® are similar; they constitute proof of a commitment to excellence. Holding Magnet Recognition is an important and influen-tial designation.

Other examples of little p include evidence-based practice guidelines and expert opinion reports generated by pro-fessional associations. These might not be thought of as policy, but their reach can be significant. Moreover, if their recom-mendations are followed across the na-tion or the globe, they are likely to have an impact on the health of populations.

Expert opinion is relegated to the bottom tier of the evidence pyramid. However, reports such as those gener-ated by the National Acad-emy of Medicine (formerly the Institute of Medicine) are credible and often contain within them systematic re-views of the literature, meta-analyses, and other catego-ries of higher-tier evidence

They are not enforceable as law, but they are, in and of themselves, extraordinarily influential.

It is also possible for a government agency or department to generate little p but as a document that is not intended to have the force and effect of law. For example, the CDC has published a number of infection control guidelines (CDC, 2017). These guidelines suggest best practices—for example, hand hygiene guidelines—but if someone fails to follow them, there are no legal consequences.

Occasionally, regulatory agencies publish opinion papers or white papers that are intended to inform or guide but that are different from law or regulation. However, in most cases, state regulatory agencies are required by their state to consider any guidance as an extension of the legislative intent in their statutes and file that information as a regulation—bringing it back into the silo of big P.

In concept, health policies—whether big P or little p—seek to address issues in health or healthcare in some way. What differs is their source (government versus private), their scope of implementation (the governmental level—for example, federal, state or local—versus the private sector), and whether the policy has the force and effect of law. Whereas failing to follow a big P could result in a range of consequences from loss of licensure to conviction of a crime, the consequences of failing to follow a little p depend entirely on the purpose and scope of the policy and the power and authority of the organization that generated the policy.

Politics in Health Policymaking

Any discussion about policymaking must also include a discussion of politics. Health policymaking occurs in a political climate; therefore, politics is inherent in the process. *Politics* is defined as "the actions or activities concerned with achieving and using power in a country or society" (Politics, n.d.) or "the science of government [or] the art or practice of administering public affairs" (Black, n.d.-b). Both of these definitions are descriptive and nonjudgmental (noting the art, science, and practice) but also carry meaning associated with power and hierarchy. Partisan politics and stakeholder influence affect the shaping of health policy and cannot be avoided or ignored.

Political Parties

Two political parties dominate US politics: the Republican party and the Democratic party. In addition, there are a varying number of smaller third parties. The two largest of these are the Libertarian party and the Green party.

Although political parties are not designated in the Constitution, they emerged almost immediately after the country was founded and have been present ever since. Each party sets its own rules, has its own platform, and elects its own leaders. Elected officials usually identify with one of the two major parties, and independents and third-party members have difficulty being heard unless they work with one of these major parties (Riaz & Akbar, 2017).

The majority party is determined by which party holds the greatest proportion of seats in each house in the US Congress. The same is true in the case of the state legislatures. Majority party control can change after each election, and the threat of change can influence what can be accomplished in each two-year congressional session or state legislature general assembly (also called a session). Therefore, elections matter in politics at the federal, state, and local level.

Except in a few states, including New Jersey and Virginia, and in a few cities, including New York City, general elections are held in November of even-numbered years. If more than one candidate from the same political party seeks election to the same office, a primary election occurs before the general election to choose which nominee from that party will advance to the general election. The timing of these primary elections varies from state to state.

A variation on the primary election is the run-off system, during which all candidates for an office run in one election. Unless one candidate gets more than half the votes, the top two candidates then face each other in a run-off election to decide who wins the office (Melhado, 2006).

Each party elects its own leadership in the House and Senate. The leaders of the majority party are powerful individuals. Party leaders designate committee leadership and make committee appointments. They also set the general agenda for the entire chamber. It is customary for party leaders to press their members to vote along party lines (depending on the significance of a particular issue). However, it is important to remember that not all members of a party may think alike. For example, even though one party may be in control of both houses of Congress or of a state legislature, members of that party might not always agree or have the same overall philosophy (Riaz & Akbar, 2017).

Stakeholders and Lobbyists

Stakeholder is a political science and government term used to describe people and groups with a direct interest in an issue. A stakeholder is generally defined as a person who has a stake in an enterprise or is involved in or affected by a course of action (Stakeholder, n.d.). In health policymaking, a stakeholder is someone with a direct or close indirect interest in a health policy area.

In nursing, we consider licensees—for example, persons licensed as RNs or APRNs—to be stakeholders with regard to the laws (nurse practice acts) and rules (regulations) that regulate their practice. The term is similarly applied to physicians and other healthcare professionals. Therefore, nurses, physicians, and other healthcare providers may be considered individual stakeholders. Nurses and other healthcare professionals may also serve as stakeholders when they are advocating for policy to protect the interests of patients they serve. (Speaking of citizens who may be patients, they also constitute a category of stakeholders.)

Additionally, the professional organizations to which nurses and other health-care professionals belong, and which represent them in policymaking arenas, are considered to be single stakeholders. For example, a nursing or medical as-sociation is considered a stakeholder. Hospital associations, long-term care as-sociations, and associations representing the pharmaceutical industry, or even retail industries in which some healthcare services such as urgent care clinics and retail pharmacies reside, are also examples of single stakeholders.

A factor worth considering is the size and political capital of a stakeholder group. A special interest group with a large membership and an ability to make significant financial contributions to political campaigns will enjoy great-er political capital. This greater political capital results in power and influence and an enhanced ability to leverage policy agendas with both elected officials and the staff of regulatory agencies charged with carrying out health policy.

Stakeholders with financial resources may also employ the services of paid professionals, called *lobbyists,* to negotiate with governmental bodies on their behalf. Career lobbyists become what are known as *stable actors.* Many have worked in government as former legislative aides or sometimes in high-level staff positions. Some are former legislators themselves. If they are straightforward with public officials and can demonstrate credibility and trustworthiness in the information they provide and the relationships they develop, legislators will seek their counsel on bills and other measures under consideration. While it is legislators' policymaking duty to conduct their own due diligence on legislative matters, their requirement to meet the needs of constituents, raise funds, and campaign can be overwhelming. Trusted interest group lobbyists can be seen as valued resources (Ozymy & Rey, 2011).

Although every person *should* take an interest in the making and carrying out of effective government health policy, this is likely an unrealistic expectation. Not everyone is comfortable with, or capable of, serving in the role of health policy advocate. However, I make this assertion because at some time, every person will have need of a nurse or other healthcare professional. Therefore, in some way, everyone may be thought of as a stakeholder in the creation of good health policy.

> The term *lobbyist* is said to have originated with President Ulysses S. Grant, who often went to a Washington, DC, hotel to escape the crowds at the White House. Even there, however, Grant found himself under siege, as representatives of special interest groups frequently stopped him in the hotel lobby to talk about their concerns (Ozymy & Rey, 2011).

Nurses and Health Policy

Health policy affects many aspects of a nurse's professional life, including the field of nursing as a whole, patients, reimbursement, tort reform, the development and use of pharmaceuticals, the design of durable medical equipment, insurance, and more (Craig, 2018). It is therefore incumbent upon nurses to take an interest and active part in health policymaking.

A recent Gallup poll shows that, for the 16th straight year, nursing is the most trusted profession (Brenan, 2017). Clearly, nurses are highly regarded by the public. The obvious question, then, is why aren't nurses more involved in health policymaking?

It seems that nurses tend to remain relatively uninvolved because they do not think they can have an impact and because they lack the confidence to articulate a health policy problem. Moreover, nurses tend to focus on differences rather than shared interests with regard to related professions (Norman & Strømseng Sjetne, 2017). This makes it difficult for many nurses to build the kind of interprofessional bridges necessary to engage in dialogue with stakeholders from other professions to advance complex health policy. Finally, the activity of policymaking is not widely promoted by the nursing profession as a whole (Anderson, Bruce, Edwards, & Podham, 2016).

Participation among nurses in health policymaking must become the norm rather than the exception. The profession must promote engagement in the political arena to identify and capitalize on political opportunities that present themselves. It must engage as a whole for our next cadre of nurses to be a part of this change.

To develop the skill set needed to effectively contribute to health policymaking, nurses must develop better leadership, communication, negotiation, and diplomacy skills, as well as increased assertiveness. Nurses must also establish the necessary connections within the health policymaking structure to enable effective change to occur (Rains & Carroll, 2000). Finally, nurses must engage as colleagues. They need to share knowledge and experiences with nurses and other healthcare providers with whom they work and collaborate. The importance of health policy development is something nurses can relate to.

Nurses can and should lead in the health policymaking arena. To do this, they must recognize policy problems that underlie many aspects of care. Gaining this recognition, and the knowledge, skills, and attitudes required to take action, should begin at the undergraduate education level (O'Neill, 2016).

One way to begin involvement in policymaking is at the organizational (little p) level. Policymaking at this level is more accessible to more people than public policymaking (big P). This is true for several reasons:

- Nurses and other healthcare providers understand the policy problems inherent in their organizations and often have a sense of workplace politics.
- These providers have a vested interest in solving policy problems.
- Organizational policymaking often results in progress, which provides a sense of accomplishment and pride in having served the organization.

- Public policymaking generally takes longer than private policymaking (Diermeier, 2009)—often two or more state legislative cycles or congressional sessions.

- Citizens and nongovernmental organizations may be at a disadvantage in the governmental policymaking sphere without the resources and influence of large corporations (including paid lobbyists).

- Public policymaking efforts are often blocked by opposing stakeholders. Because lobbying for government reform takes more time than volunteers representing professional organizations can offer, well-funded corporate interests can easily counter-lobby (Baron & Diermeier, 2007; Diermeier, 2009).

In addition to increasing participation in policymaking in the workplace, nurses should increase participation in government policymaking. However, government policymaking is best accomplished in association with one's professional organizations. Nurses need to do more than simply join these professional organizations, however (although this is a good start); they must engage with and contribute their unique gifts to the organization. Through engagement, nurses can challenge old ways of doing things, in policy and practice.

The notion that nurses should be involved in making health policy is not new. Indeed, health policymaking is a part of nursing's history. Many nursing organizations in the US have published statements about member engagement in health policymaking. This engagement has become an integral professional expectation and is reflected in the American Nurses Association Code of Ethics for Nurses with Interpretive Statements (2015).

> One of the first steps toward change is for nurses to become better informed about health policymaking structures and processes and about the wise use of evidence to advance nursing's policy agenda.

Chaos Theory, the Butterfly Effect, and the Charge to Advance Health Policy Change

Chaos theory, which is based on mathematical models, focuses on the behavior of dynamic systems that are highly sensitive to some particular initiating condition and has been adapted to explain human situations involving chaos, uncertainty, and complexity, including choice-making in the policy arena (Sa, 2004). The notion of complex adaptive systems has also been used to describe the increasingly complex healthcare system (Plsek & Greenhalgh, 2001).

Embedded in chaos theory is a phenomenon called the *butterfly effect.* It pertains to *fractals,* which are never-ending patterns. The butterfly effect is based on the idea that in a complex system, a minute change at a local level at a point in time can have large effects elsewhere in the system at a later point in time. Scientists illustrate this effect by suggesting that a butterfly flapping its wings at the right point in space and time in a particular geographical location could have the effect of causing a hurricane at a later point in space and time halfway across the globe (Fractal Foundation, n.d.; Oestreicher, 2007). The butterfly effect can be applied to describe how small-scale events at one point in time can drive and influence larger-scale outcomes at a later point in time. Much of what occurs in politics and the policymaking environment is initiated on a small scale or driven by smaller groups, but the effects are often felt on a much larger scale!

When they engage as a unified voice in the political and policymaking process, nurses and other healthcare providers can become a force similar to what is envisioned at the point in time when the butterfly flaps its wings. What can seem like a small effort at one point in time might drive significant outcomes at a later point in time. By playing a part in the process, they can help to advance good health policy and ultimately make a difference for their practice and the patients they serve.

Summary

This chapter defined, described, and differentiated key terms related to health policy, including policy, public policy, and health policy. It also discussed the relationship between health policy—particularly public health policy—and the health of populations. It presented health policy as both an entity and a process.

As noted in this chapter, policy is generated by both governments (big P) and private organizations (little P). The former has the force and effect of law, and the latter does not—although policy generated by private organizations can be both important and influential.

The chapter went on to discuss the role politics plays in health policymaking and examined the nature of stakeholders and lobbyists in the process. It ended by examining potential contributions by nurses and other healthcare professionals to policymaking and exhorting them to engage in the process to advance health policy.

References

American Nurses Association. (2015). Code of Ethics for Nurses with Interpretive Statements. Retrieved from https://www.nursingworld.org/practice-policy/nursing-excellence/ethics/code-of-ethics-for-nurses/

Anderson, J., Bruce, B., Edwards, M., & Podham, M. (2016). Engaging rural nurses in the policy development process. *Contemporary Nurse, 52*(6), 677–685. doi:10.1080/10376178.2016.1221323

Apollonio, D. E., & Bero, L. A. (2016). Challenges to generating evidence-informed policy and the role of systematic reviews and (perceived) conflicts of interest. *Journal of Communication in Healthcare, 9*(2), 135–141. doi:10.1080/17538068.2016.1182784

Baron, D. P., & Diermeier, D. (2007). Strategic activism and nonmarket strategy. *Journal of Economics & Management Strategy, 16*(3), 599–634. doi:10.1111/j.1530-9134.2007.00152.x

Black, H. C. (n.d.-a). Policy. In *Black's Law Dictionary,* 2nd ed. Retrieved from https://thelawdictionary.org/policy/

Black, H. C. (n.d.-b). Politics. In *Black's Law Dictionary,* 2nd ed. Retrieved from https://thelawdictionary.org/politics/

Black, H. C. (n.d.-c). Public policy. In *Black's Law Dictionary,* 2nd ed. Retrieved from https://thelawdictionary.org/public-policy/

Black, H. C. (n.d.-d). State. In *Black's Law Dictionary,* 2nd ed. Retrieved from https://thelawdictionary.org/state-n/

Brenan, M. (2017, Dec. 26). Nurses keep healthy lead as most honest, ethical profession. *Gallup.* Retrieved from https://news.gallup.com/poll/224639/nurses-keep-healthy-lead-honest-ethical-profession.aspx

Centers for Disease Control and Prevention. (2015). CDC policy process. Retrieved from https://www.cdc.gov/policy/analysis/process/index.html

Centers for Disease Control and Prevention. (2017). Infection control: Guidelines library. Retrieved from https://www.cdc.gov/infectioncontrol/guidelines/index.html

Craig, G. (2018). What does health policy mean to nursing? *American Nurse Today, 13*(5), 37.

Diermeier, D. (2009). *Governing the global economy: The role of private politics.* Volume 40 of working paper series. Policy Research Initiative.

Easton, D. (1953). *The political system: An inquiry into the state of political science.* New York, NY: Knopf.

Fractal Foundation. (n.d.). What is chaos theory? Retrieved from https://fractalfoundation.org/resources/what-is-chaos-theory/

Hlavac, J., Beagley, J., & Zucchi, E. (2018). Applications of policy and the advancement of patients' health outcomes through interpreting services: Data and viewpoints from a major public healthcare provider. *Translation & Interpreting, 10*(1), 111–136. doi:10.12807/ti.110201.2018.a07

Latham, S. R. (2018). Sunset law: Statute. *Encyclopedia Britannica.* Retrieved from https://www.britannica.com/topic/sunset-law

Longest, B. B. (1998). *Health policymaking in the United States* (2nd ed.). Ann Arbor, MI: Association of University Programs in Health Administration/Health Administration Press (AUPHA/HAP).

Melhado, E. M. (2006). Health planning in the United States and the decline of public-interest policymaking. *Milbank Quarterly, 84*(2), 359–440. doi:10.1111/j.1468-0009.2006.00451.x

Norman, R. M., & Strømseng Sjetne, I. (2017). Measuring nurses' perception of work environment: A scoping review of questionnaires. *BMC Nursing, 16,* 1–15. doi:10.1186/s12912-017-0256-9

Oestreicher, C. (2007). A history of chaos theory. *Dialogues in Clinical Neuroscience, 9*(3), 279–289.

O'Neill, M. (2016). Policy-focused service-learning as a capstone: Teaching essentials of baccalaureate nursing education. *Journal of Nursing Education, 55*(10), 583–586. doi:10.3928/01484834-20160914-08

Ozymy, J., & Rey, D. (2011). Legislative ambition, resources, and lobbyist influence in U.S. state legislatures. *The Journal of Political Science, 39,* 33–53.

Pacheco, J., & Boushey, G. (2014). Public health and agenda setting: Determinants of state attention to tobacco and vaccines. *Journal of Health Politics, Policy & Law, 39*(3), 565–589. doi:10.1215/03616878-2682612

Plsek, P. E., & Greenhalgh, T. (2001). The challenge of complexity in health care. *British Medical Journal, 323*(7313), 625–628. doi:10.1136/bmj.323.7313.625

Politics. (n.d.). In *Collins English dictionary.* Retrieved from https://www.collinsdictionary.com/us/dictionary/english/politics

Public policy. (n.d.). In *Merriam-Webster's online dictionary.* Retrieved from https://www.merriam-webster.com/dictionary/public%20policy

Rains, J. W., & Carroll, K. L. (2000). The effect of health policy education on self-perceived political assessment of graduate nursing students. *Journal of Nursing Education, 39,* 37–40.

Riaz, A., & Akbar, M. (2017). Ideologies of US political parties and their influence on domestic issues of America. *Pakistan Journal of Social Sciences, 37*(1), 231–240.

Sa, D. W. (2004). Chaos, uncertainty, and policy choice: Utilizing the adaptive model. *International Review of Public Administration, 8*(2), 119–128. doi:10.1080/12294659.2004.10805034

Semanskee, A., Levitt, L., & Cox, C. (2018). Data note: Changes in enrollment in the individual health insurance market. *Henry J Kaiser Family Foundation*. Retrieved from https://www.kff.org/health-reform/issue-brief/data-note-changes-in-enrollment-in-the-individual-health-insurance-market/

Shi, L. (2013). *Introduction to health policy* (1st ed.). Chicago, IL: Health Administration Press.

Stakeholder. (n.d.). In *Merriam-Webster's online dictionary*. Retrieved from https://www.merriam-webster.com/dictionary/stakeholder

US National Library of Medicine. (2004). Collection development manual: Health policy. Retrieved from https://www.nlm.nih.gov/tsd/acquisitions/cdm/subjects45.html

World Health Organization. (2018). Health topics: Health policy. Retrieved from http://www.who.int/topics/health_policy/en/

"The only sure bulwark of continuing liberty is a government strong enough to protect the interests of the people, and a people strong enough and well enough informed to maintain its sovereign control over the government."

–Franklin D. Roosevelt

4

GOVERNMENT STRUCTURES AND FUNCTIONS THAT DRIVE PROCESS

–JACQUELINE M. LOVERSIDGE, PHD, RNC-AWHC
JOYCE ZURMEHLY, PHD, DNP, RN, NEA-BC, ANEF

KEY CONTENT IN THIS CHAPTER

- The three branches of government
- The legislative branch: the Senate and the House of Representatives
- The executive branch: the offices of the president and vice president and the cabinet
- The judicial branch: the Supreme Court and federal courts
- The structure and function of state governments
- The structure and function of executive branch agencies and regulatory boards

The Three Branches of Government

The American government follows a federal model consisting of three branches, independent of one another, each with its own scope of authority. These branches are as follows (USA.gov, 2018):

- **Legislative:** This branch makes laws. The legislative branch in the US federal government consists of two chambers: the Senate and the House of Representatives. Collectively, these two chambers are referred to as Congress.

- **Executive:** This branch implements and enforces laws. The head of the executive branch is the president.

- **Judicial:** This branch evaluates and interprets laws. This branch consists of three tiers of courts of law, with the Supreme Court at the top.

This structure provides for a balance of power; that is, it ensures that no one branch will have more power or authority than the others. This balance of power is established in the Constitution of the United States, which was, and continues to be, designed to provide for a strong yet flexible government that meets the needs of the republic and protects its citizens' rights and freedoms (Supreme Court of the US, n.d.-b).

To ensure this balance of power, each branch has distinct and separate responsibilities. These responsibilities serve as a series of checks and balances. Checks and balances in the system include the following:

- The legislative branch creates laws, but for the laws to be enacted, they must be signed by the president, who is the head of the executive branch. The president can veto bills, but a veto may be overridden by a two-thirds vote by each chamber in the legislature (US Senate, n.d.-c).

- The president appoints (nominates) federal judges and Supreme Court justices. However, the Senate must affirm them (UShistory.org, 2018).

- The legislature, with the signature of the president, may enact laws, and the president may enact executive actions (orders). However, the Supreme Court may invalidate any law or executive order after a procedure of judicial review if, in the court's judgment, the law conflicts with the US Constitution (Supreme Court of the US, n.d.-b).

- Setting the federal budget is a complicated process that requires involvement of both the executive branch and the legislative branch. The congressional budget process begins when the president releases his or her proposal for a budget resolution, the main purpose of which is to develop a framework for Congress. The president's budget resolution is compiled, prepared, and submitted by the Office of Management and Budget, which is part of the executive branch. Committees in both the House and the Senate are responsible for passing budget resolutions and appropriations bills. To achieve this, committee members must consider revenue, spending, a spending limit, and other budget issues. The appropriations bills and the budget in their final forms are signed by the president (Budget House Committee, 2018; National Conference of State Legislatures, n.d.).

> The governments of 49 of the 50 states comprising the United States are structured similarly to the federal model. One state has a single house. You'll learn more about state governments later in this chapter.

The Legislative Branch: The Senate and the House of Representatives

The legislative branch of the federal government is seen as the branch of government closest to the people. This branch is *bicameral*. That is, it consists of two chambers: the Senate and the House of Representatives (Hakim, 2007). The two chambers are structured differently, and each has its own organization and rules.

Both chambers make use of committees. Of these there are three main types:

- **Standing committees:** These are permanent committees. Standing committees consider bills and issues and make recommendations to their full, respective chambers. Standing committees also have oversight responsibility and may monitor programs, activities, and government agencies within their jurisdiction. They recommend funding levels, known as *authorizations,* for government operations and for new or existing programs. Other functions are committee-specific. Standing committees are identified in their respective chamber rules (Senate Rule XXV and House Rule X).

- **Select or special committees:** These are established by a resolution of the chamber. They might conduct investigations or studies, or could be convened to consider certain legislative measures. Some select or special committees examine emerging issues that do not fit cleanly into standing committee jurisdictions. A select or special committee can be established on a permanent or temporary basis and may restrict membership to certain specified representatives. (Note that the Senate is more likely to use the term *special committee*.)

- **Joint committees:** These consist of members from both the House and the Senate. Permanent joint committees generally perform housekeeping tasks or conduct studies rather than consider measures such as bills. Chairmanship usually alternates between a member of the House and a member of the Senate. A *conference committee* is a type of temporary joint committee that forms only to resolve differences between competing House and Senate versions of a measure, such as a bill. The compromise drafted by the conference committee is submitted to the full House and Senate, which must approve the compromise for the measure to move on (Heitshusen, 2017).

> Other types of committees, such as party committees, task forces, and organizations of congressional members, are informal in nature.

The Senate

The US Constitution called for the creation of the Senate in 1787. The Senate was modeled after the governors' councils of the colonial era and the various state senates that evolved following independence. The Senate has a long and fascinating history. Although the structure and function of the Senate has changed somewhat since its first session convened in March 1789, much has remained the same.

The framers of the US Constitution agreed that each state should be represented equally in the Senate, with two senators per state. Currently, the Senate consists of 100 members—two for each of the 50 states in the Union. In its early years, state legislatures selected the US senators for their state. However, after state legislatures repeatedly deadlocked during this process, federal legislators passed the 17th Amendment to the US Constitution in 1913, which provided for direct popular election of US senators (US Senate, n.d.-f).

The Constitution also sets forth minimal qualifications, term lengths, and term rotations for US senators. As for qualifications, US senators must be at least 30 years old, must have been a citizen of the US for nine years, and must be a resident of the state he or she represents. The term of office for a senator is six years. Approximately one-third of the total membership of the Senate is elected every two years; in this way, only one-third of serving members are junior members (US Senate, n.d.-i). The three divisions, or thirds, are designated by Article I, Section 2 of the Constitution as classes.

Leadership and officers of the Senate are established by the Constitution and by political parties. Two leaders are mandated by the Constitution. The primary Senate leader is the vice president of the US. The second is the president pro tempore. The Constitution does not call for the establishment of political party leaders; these emerged during the 20th century. Both Republican and Democratic floor leaders are elected by their party at the beginning of each two-year congressional session and represent their party's positions on political issues. One serves as a majority leader and the other as a minority leader, depending on which party holds the majority of Senate seats. The majority leader has a powerful role. He or she schedules the daily program of legislation and establishes agreement on the time for debate. The majority party leaders open Senate proceedings and keep the business of the Senate flowing. Both majority and minority party leaders keep legislation moving when they are able and protect party members' rights. In addition to the majority leader and the minority leader, there are a number of other, lesser leadership positions (US Senate, n.d.-d).

The Senate employs a staff that supports the work of senators (US Senate, n.d.-e). One such staff member is the secretary of the Senate, an officer of the Senate elected by the Senate members (US Senate, n.d.-g) who plays an important operational role in the oversight of legislative, financial, and administrative functions. The secretary of the Senate supervises an extensive list of services and offices responsible for daily operations, including the Senate clerks, curators, IT, payroll disbursement, Senate page education, and public record maintenance. Other Senate staff members include a sergeant at arms, senate chaplains, and party secretaries (US Senate, n.d.-e).

Senate committees conduct much of the Senate's business. Because the work is so complex and because there is so much of it, there are at present 20 permanent committees and 4 joint committees (see Table 4.1). Of the 20 permanent committees, 16 are standing committees; these are permanent bodies and have specific responsibilities according to the Senate's official rules. Four are special or select committees; these were created for specific purposes and may not have been considered permanent when they were created (US Senate, n.d.-h). However, they have become permanent over time and are listed among the 20 permanent committees (US Senate, n.d.-b).

In addition, temporary committees are occasionally established. Although the Senate has set guidelines for committees, individual committees often adopt committee-specific rules and procedures. Parties play an important part in Senate committees. Committee chairs represent the majority party and set the committee's agenda. Parties also establish membership of senators on committees. Committee business includes the consideration of bills and resolutions, which might be managed by the committee's chair through the full Senate's deliberation. Committees also handle the confirmation or rejection of presidential nominees, such as Supreme Court justices. Finally, they consider treaties, hold international hearings, might hold oversight hearings, and can initiate investigations of wrongdoing if suspected (US Senate, n.d.-b).

TABLE 4.1   US Senate Committees

Permanent Committees		Joint Committees
Agriculture, Nutrition, and Forestry	Health, Education, Labor, and Pensions	Joint Committee on Printing
Appropriations	Homeland Seecurity and Government Affairs	Joint Committee on Taxation
Armed Services		Joint Committee on the Library
Banking, Housing, and Urban Affairs	Indian Affairs (Select Committee)	Joint Economic Committee
Budget	Judiciary	
Commerce, Science, and Transportation	Rules and Administration	
Energy and Natural Resources	Select Committee on Ethics	
Environment and Public Works	Select Committee on Intelligence	
Finance	Small Business and Entrepreneurship	
Foreign Relations	Special Committee on Aging	
	Veterans' Affairs	

US Senate, n.d.-b

Senators also organize informally into groups, without official recognition, called Senate *caucuses*. These informal groups consist of members with shared interests in specific issues or philosophies. Caucuses have been part of the policymaking process in the US since colonial times. Only one Senate caucus is officially recognized: the Senate Caucus on International Narcotics Control, which was established by law in 1985 (US Senate, n.d.-a).

The House of Representatives

The US House of Representatives is considered the lower house in Congress. This is because it structurally resembles the British House of Commons of Parliament more closely than the House of Lords (which is known as the *upper house*). It is closer to the people in that its members represent the citizens of their states according to population. It is the only branch of the federal government whose members have been elected directly by the citizenry since its founding in 1789 (US House of Representatives: History, Art & Archives, n.d.-b). Members of the US House are called *representatives*. A representative may also be referred to as a *congressman* or *congresswoman*.

The number of voting representatives in the House is established by law. It is fixed at no more than 435 members, representing the population of all 50 states. Whereas senators serve an entire state, representatives serve the people of a specific congressional district. Districts are redrawn every decade based on population data gathered by the US Census. In addition to state representatives, one delegate also currently represents each of the following: the District of Columbia (DC), the US Virgin Islands, Guam, American Samoa, and the Commonwealth of the Northern Mariana Islands. Delegates participate differently in Congress from representatives. For example, the role of the delegate from DC is marginalized. This person has no vote, and his or her constituents are not represented in Congress in the same manner as the citizens of the 50 states (GovTrack, n.d.). The role of other delegates is the same as the one representing DC. Puerto Rico is represented by a resident commissioner, who has the right to debate in Congress but not vote (Rundquist, n.d.; US House of Representatives, n.d.-b).

As with the Senate, the Constitution sets forth minimal qualifications and term lengths for members of the House of Representatives. These are established in Article I, Section 2, Clause 2. The term of office for a representative is two years. A representative must be at least 25 years old, must have been a citizen of the US for seven years, and must be a resident of the state he or she represents. These qualifications are less restrictive than those for senators because the country's founders intended for the House to be the legislative chamber closest to the people (US House of Representatives: History, Art & Archives, n.d.-a).

Gerrymandering

In most states, the majority party in the state legislature controls the process for setting congressional and state legislative districts. As mentioned, this process, called *redistricting,* occurs every 10 years. The redistricting process, which uses data gathered through the US Census, is decidedly political in nature. Inevitably, the majority party attempts to draw the electoral map in a way that gives it an unfair advantage over its rival party, although some states use nonpartisan commissions to establish district lines. As a result, it is often difficult for the minority party to win—even if it receives more votes overall.

The process of drawing electoral maps in a partisan manner is called *gerrymandering* (Warrington, 2018). The term comes from the name of former Massachusetts Governor Elbridge Gerry, whose administration enacted a law defining new and advantageous state senatorial districts in 1812 (Gerrymandering, n.d.). This is occasionally done in such a way that it raises questions of constitutionality and disproportional representation (Warrington, 2018).

Leadership in the House of Representatives is determined by members of the majority and minority parties. (Third parties generally do not have sufficient numbers to elect their own leaders, and independents usually ally with one of the major parties.) The primary leader, called the *speaker of the House,* is elected by the House of Representatives as a whole. The speaker—who is an elected representative from his or her state district—serves as the presiding officer and administrative head of the House and is second in the line of presidential succession after the vice president (US House of Representatives, n.d.-c). By tradition, the speaker is elected from the majority caucus, but it is not required that the speaker be a member of the majority party. Article I, Section 2, Clause 5 of the US Constitution mandates the office of speaker of the House, but the House and individual speakers have molded the position over time (US House of Representatives Office of the Historian, n.d.).

The speaker is in the position of highest authority over the body of the House of Representatives and, as such, is the leader for the majority party of the House. In addition to the speaker, House positions include the majority leader, who represents the majority party on the House floor, and the minority leader, who represents the minority party on the House floor. These positions are not mandated by the US Constitution but have been established over time and are controlled by the majority and minority caucuses, respectively. Additionally, as in the Senate, there are other, lesser party leadership roles for House members of both parties (US House of Representatives, n.d.-c).

The House of Representatives is staffed by a number of officers and in-house organizations, which support the legislative work of congressional members and committee offices. Officers and organizations of the House include a chaplain, a chief administrative officer, a clerk of the House, a general counsel, a historian, an inspector general, the Office of Congressional Ethics, the Office of the Law Revision Counsel, the Office of the Legislative Counsel, a parliamentarian of the House, and a sergeant at arms (US House of Representatives, n.d.-d).

The House of Representative divides its work among 21 permanent committees, which consider bills and issues and oversee issues, programs, and activities that fall within their jurisdiction, and two joint select committees (see Table 4.2). Members of the House also serve on the four joint select committees identified in Table 4.1 (US House of Representatives, n.d.-a).

TABLE 4.2   US House of Representatives Committees

Permanent Committees		Join Select Committees
Agriculture	Natural Resources	Joint Select Committee on Budget and Appropriations Process Reform
Appropriations	Oversight and Government Reform	
Armed Services		
Budget	Permanent Select Committee on Intelligence	
Education and the Workforce		Joint Select Committee on Solvency of Multiemployer Pension Plans
Energy and Commerce	Rules	
Ethics	Science, Space, and Technology	
Financial Services	Small Business	
Foreign Affairs	Transportation and Infrastructure	
Homeland Security		
House Administration	Veterans' Affairs	
Judiciary	Ways and Means	

Like the Senate, members of the House of Representatives also organize themselves into caucuses or conferences. Some of these are centered around philosophical orientations—for example, consisting of conservative, liberal or centrist, or progressive Democrats, or conservative or moderate Republicans. Others are composed of members of a particular race or ethnic group. Still others consist of bipartisan members unified around a special interest. Rules for forming these organizations—of which there are several; a 2017 list runs some 50 pages—are established by the Committee on House Administration (Committee on House Administration, n.d.-a, n.d.-b).

The Executive Branch: The Offices of the President and Vice President and the Cabinet

The executive branch of the federal government is responsible for implementing and enforcing the laws written by Congress. The power of this branch is vested in the president of the US, who, under Article II of the Constitution, acts as both head of state and commander in chief of the armed forces. Second in command in the executive branch is the vice president, who assumes the presidency if the need arises (The White House, n.d.-a).

Presidential powers include the authority to:

- Sign legislation enacted by Congress into law
- Veto bills that have been enacted by Congress (note that Congress can override a presidential veto with a two-thirds vote in both chambers)
- Negotiate and sign treaties (these must be ratified by a two-thirds vote in the Senate)
- Extend pardons and clemency for federal crimes (except in cases of impeachment)
- Issue executive orders, which direct executive officers or clarify or further existing laws (these have the force and effect of law but do not require approval by Congress; The White House, n.d.-a)
- Override or bypass Congress in times of emergency, such as in times of war

In times of emergency, the bounds of executive orders are virtually limitless (Cornell Law School, n.d.; The White House, n.d.-a). Indeed, because of the power and authority granted to the office of the president and the capacity of the president to issue executive orders, even war can be declared (Acs, 2016). Other measures can also be executed on the basis of executive order.

Because the list of presidential powers is extensive, the Constitution requires periodic reporting to Congress in the form of an address called the *State of the Union.* The president may fulfill this duty in a form of his or her choosing, but the joint congressional session State of the Union address in January has become the tradition (The White House, n.d.-a).

A complete list of executive orders issued since 1994 is available through the *Federal Register (Federal Register,* n.d.). Recent executive orders in the current administration at the time of this writing have re-imposed sanctions on Iran and established the National Council for the American Worker, the Task Force on Market Integrity and Consumer Fraud, and the Ocean Policy to Advance the Economic, Security, and Environmental Interests of the United States (*Federal Register,* n.d.).

The Constitution sets forth qualifications and term limits for the office of president. The president must be at least 35 years old, must be a natural-born citizen, and must have lived in the US for a minimum of 14 years. The president is not elected directly by the people. Rather, he or she is elected by an institution called the *Electoral College.* The Electoral College currently consists of 538 electors. These electors are apportioned according to the population in each of the 50 states. A president is limited to two four-year terms (The White House, n.d.-a).

The vice president's primary responsibility is to be ready to assume the office of the presidency should the president become unable to perform his or her duties—for example, due to death, resignation, or temporary incapacitation. In the event of the latter, the vice president and the cabinet (discussed momentarily) have the authority to judge whether the president is no longer able to fulfill his or her duties. The vice president is elected with the president by the Electoral College. The duties of the vice president, beyond those described in the Constitution, are at the discretion of the president. Vice presidents have approached the role differently throughout history (The White House, n.d.-a).

The Line of Succession

Should the president become unable to fulfill his or her duties, the line of succession is as follows: the vice president, the speaker of the House, the Senate president pro tempore, followed by members of the cabinet in the order in which their departments were created (The White House, n.d.-a).

The president's staff, as well as entities such as the Office of Management and Budget (OMB) and the Office of the US Trade Representative, are part of something called the *Executive Office of the President* (EOP). Many of the president's closest advisors work in the EOP, which is overseen by the White House chief of staff (The White House, n.d.-a). Some of these advisors require Senate confirmation, but most are appointed at the president's discretion. Staff and positions shift in the EOP as the president identifies different priorities. The current EOP employs more than 1,800 people (The White House, n.d.-a).

The *cabinet* is an advisory body comprising the heads of 15 executive departments. These and other departments and agencies carry out the day-to-day responsibilities of the executive branch and the administration and enforcement of federal laws. Table 4.3 lists executive branch cabinet departments and functions. Members of the cabinet are appointed by the president and confirmed by the Senate. Cabinet members are referred to by the title *secretary*, except for the head of the Justice Department, who is called the *attorney general*. (The attorney general [AG] represents the US in legal matters, advises the president and government executive department heads, and may appear in person before the Supreme Court.) There are also numerous executive agencies that are not part of the presidential cabinet but that fall under the president's authority and whose heads are appointed by the president. In addition, the president appoints federal judges, ambassadors, and the heads of other federal offices.

TABLE 4.3   Executive Branch Cabinet Departments and
Functions

Cabinet Department	Functions
Department of Agriculture (USDA)	Develops and executes policy on farming, agriculture, and food
	Ensures food safety
	Protects natural resources
	Provides surplus foods to developing countries
	Engages in oversees aid programs
Department of Commerce	Improves living standards by promoting economic development and technological innovation
	Supports US business and industry
	Promotes US exports
	Assists in the creation of and enforces international trade agreements
Department of Defense (DOD)	Provides the military forces needed to deter war against the US
	Protects the security of the country
	Headquartered at the Pentagon
	Includes the Army, Navy, Air Force, and other military agencies, offices, and commands
	Includes the joint chiefs of staff, Pentagon Force Protection Agency, National Security Agency, and Defense Intelligence Agency
Department of Education	Promotes student achievement and preparation for competition in a global economy
	Fosters educational excellence
	Ensures equal access to education
	Administers financial aid
	Collects data
	Complements state and local efforts

continues

TABLE 4.3 Executive Branch Cabinet Departments and Functions (cont.)

Cabinet Department	Functions
Department of Energy (DOE)	Advances national, economic, and energy security of the US
	Encourages the development of reliable, clean, affordable energy
	Ensures US nuclear security
Department of Health and Human Services (HHS)	Principal agency for protecting the health of Americans
	Provides essential human services
	Conducts health and social science research
	Prevents disease outbreaks
	Ensures food and drug safety
	Provides health insurance, including the administration of Medicare and Medicaid
	Oversees the National Institutes of Health (NIH), Federal Drug Administration (FDA), and Centers for Disease Control and Prevention (CDC)
Department of Homeland Security	Prevents and disrupts terrorist attacks and manages federal emergencies
	Protects American people, infrastructure, and key resources
	Responds to and recovers from incidents that do occur
	Established by the Homeland Security Act of 2002 after the terrorist attacks of September 11, 2001
	Consolidates 22 executive branch agencies, including the US Customs Service, US Coast Guard, US Secret Service, Transportation Security Administration, and Federal Emergency Management Agency
Department of Housing and Urban Development (HUD)	Responsible for national policies and programs to address America's housing needs
	Enforces fair housing laws
	Oversees the Federal Housing Administration (FHA), Office of Fair Housing and Equal Opportunity, and Community Development Block Grant Program
	Administers public housing and homeless assistance

Department of the Interior (DOI)	Conserves and protects America's natural resources
	Offers recreation opportunities
	Conducts scientific research
	Conserves and protects fish and wildlife
	Honors trust responsibility to American Indians, Alaskan Natives, and island communities
	Oversees the Bureau of Indian Affairs, Minerals Management Service, and US Geological Survey
	Manages national parks
	Protects endangered species
Department of Justice	Enforces the law and defends the interests of the US according to the law
	Ensures public safety against federal and domestic threats
	Provides federal leadership in preventing and controlling crime
	Seeks punishment for those guilty of breaking the law
	Oversees 40 organizations, including the Drug Enforcement Administration (DEA), Federal Bureau of Investigation (FBI), US Marshals, and Federal Bureau of Prisons
Department of Labor	Oversees federal programs to ensure a strong American workforce
	Includes programs on job training, safe working conditions, minimum hourly wage, overtime pay, employment discrimination, and unemployment insurance
	Includes the Bureau of Labor Statistics and Occupational Safety and Health Administration (OSHA)
Department of State	Facilitates the development and implementation of the president's foreign policy
	Represents the US abroad
	Provides foreign assistance and military training programs
	Counters international crime
	Supports services to US citizens and foreign nationals seeking entrance to the US
	Maintains diplomatic relations with approximately 180 countries through the deployment of civilian US Foreign Service employees

continues

TABLE 4.3 Executive Branch Cabinet Departments and Functions (cont.)

Cabinet Department	Functions
Department of Transportation (DOT)	Ensures a safe, fast, efficient, accessible, and convenient transportation system to meet vital national interests
	Includes the Federal Highway Administration, Federal Aviation Administration, National Highway Traffic Safety Administration, Federal Transit Administration, Federal Railroad Administration, and Maritime Administration
Department of the Treasury	Promotes economic prosperity
	Ensures soundness and security of US and international financial systems
	Produces coin and currency
	Disperses payments to the American public
	Collects taxes
	Borrows funds as necessary to run the federal government
	Ensures national security by improving safeguards to financial systems and implementing economic sanctions against foreign threats to the US
Department of Veterans Affairs	Administers benefit programs for veterans, families, and their survivors (about 25% of the nation's population are potentially eligible)
	Benefits include pension, education, disability compensation, home loans, life insurance, vocational rehabilitation, survivor support, medical care, and burial benefits

The White House, n.d.-a

Sometimes, multiple cabinet-level departments are involved in a single domain. For example, consider the domain of health. One cabinet-level department, the Department of Health and Human Services, focuses solely on this domain, while several others are connected to it indirectly. For example:

- The education of nurses and other health professions falls under the purview of the Department of Education.
- The Department of Labor oversees workplace health and safety.

- The Department of State oversees diplomatic relations, which has an impact on global health.
- The Department of Veterans Affairs oversees the care of veterans.

The Judicial Branch: The Supreme Court and Federal Courts

Article III of the Constitution establishes the judicial branch of the federal government. Article III, Section 1 states that "The judicial Power of the United States, shall be vested in one supreme Court, and in such inferior Courts as the Congress may from time to time ordain and establish" (US Courts, n.d.-a). Although the Constitution establishes that there should be a Supreme Court of the US, it is left to Congress to determine how that court will be organized.

The highest court in the land, the Supreme Court is the "court of last resort" for those seeking justice. It plays a significant role in the constitutional system of government. It has the power of judicial review, which ensures a balance of power among the branches of government, and it protects civil rights and liberties by striking down laws in violation of the US Constitution. Although the federal judiciary is a separate branch of government, it often works with the executive and legislative branches as the Constitution requires (Supreme Court of the US, n.d.-b; US Courts, n.d.-b).

There are qualifications, procedures for appointment, and term considerations for Supreme Court justices. The Constitution does not specify that a justice must be a lawyer, but all justices must have been trained in the law. All federal justices—including Supreme Court justices—are appointed by the president and confirmed by the Senate by a simple majority vote.

Currently, there is one chief justice and eight associate justices on the Supreme Court (US Courts, n.d.-a). There is no requirement that the chief justice serve first as an associate justice, but many have done so. There is no term limit for justices specified in the Constitution, which states that justices "shall hold their Offices during good Behaviour." This means that a justice may hold office for life should he or she choose to do so and can be removed only by the impeachment process (Supreme Court of the US, n.d.-a).

The jurisdiction of the Supreme Court—its legal ability to hear a case—is established in Article III, Section 2 of the Constitution. The court may have jurisdiction to try certain cases—for example, suits between two or more states and/or cases involving ambassadors or other public officials. The court also has *appellate jurisdiction*—that is, the court can hear appeals. Appeals can be heard on almost any case that concerns a point involving constitutional and/or federal law. When exercising its appellate jurisdiction, the court does not have to hear the case but can review the case instead. The court also has the power of *judicial review,* by which it can declare a legislative or executive act in violation of the Constitution. This power is essential in ensuring that the legislative and executive branches of government recognize the limits of their power (US Courts, n.d.-a).

Lower courts in the federal court system sit below the Supreme Court. These include 94 district courts, which are organized into 12 circuits, or districts (hence their name). District courts are trial courts. That is, they apply legal principles to resolve disputes. Every state has at least one district court. There is also a district court in the District of Columbia and in each of the four US territories. In addition to the 94 district courts, there are 13 courts of appeals—one for each of the 12 districts, plus a 13th circuit, which is the Federal Judicial Circuit. The Federal Judicial Circuit has nationwide jurisdiction but hears only certain appeals depending on subject matter (USLegal, 2016). The role of these appellate courts is to determine whether the law was applied correctly at the district-court level. Appeals courts each consist of three judges with no jury. The courts of appeals hear challenges to district-court decisions from within their circuit as well as appeals from decisions regarding federal administrative agencies.

In addition to district and appellate courts, there is a US bankruptcy court, which has jurisdiction over bankruptcy cases. There are also three legislative courts—the US Court of Appeals for Veterans Claims, the US Court of Appeals for the Armed Forces, and the US Tax Court—created by Congress under Article I of the Constitution. These courts do not have full judicial power; rather, their authority is limited to questions of Constitutional law (US Courts, n.d.-b).

The Structure and Function of State and Local Governments

The 10th Amendment of the Constitution establishes that "the powers not delegated to the United States by the Constitution, nor prohibited by it to the states, are reserved to the states respectively, or to the people" (The Heritage Guide to the Constitution, 2017). The governments of all 50 states are modeled after the federal government. As such, they consist of the same three branches—executive, legislative, and judicial—although this model is not required, and states may organize as they see fit.

Every state's executive branch is headed by a governor, who is elected by the people. Other state executive branch leaders are also directly elected by the people and may include a lieutenant governor, attorney general, secretary of state, auditors, and commissioners (The White House, n.d.-b). The length of gubernatorial terms and term limits varies by state. Some are established within the state constitution, while others have been created through various initiatives (Ballotpedia, n.d.-c). The power of the governor's office depends on the state. In some states, the governor initiates the state budget process. Some governors have line-item veto power over legislative measures in addition to full veto power. *Line-item veto power* has the effect of allowing a governor to selectively veto sections of a bill deemed not in the best interest of the state or its citizens. This is especially important for legislation such as budget bills. In most states, the legislature can override a line-item veto by a two-thirds vote.

Governors' cabinets consist of the heads of various state-level departments. How cabinet members are appointed and confirmed, and which departments hold cabinet-level status, is established by each state's constitution. Additional executive branch agencies include noncabinet-level state agencies and regulatory boards, such as boards that regulate various professions. Regulation of professions is an example of powers that are not within the purview of the federal government and are instead reserved for the state. Professional practice acts include those regulating nursing, medicine, pharmacy, counselors and social workers, architects, engineers, funeral directors and embalmers, and cosmetologists, to name just a few. All these exist in state, not federal, law. (This is why a federal nurse practice act that would enable easy state-to-state mobility is not possible.)

Each of the 50 states has a legislature composed of elected officials. The legislature considers matters brought to it by the governor or introduced by its members. This body creates legislation (which is signed into law by the state's governor), approves the state's budget, initiates tax legislation, and may initiate articles of impeachment in a way that mirrors the federal system of checks and balances. And, like the federal government, state legislatures are bicameral, with a smaller upper chamber (a senate) and a larger lower chamber (a house of representatives or house of delegates). (One exception is Nebraska, which has a *unicameral* legislature—that is, it consists of only one chamber.) Members of the upper chamber generally serve longer terms than those of the lower chamber, with senators usually serving four-year terms and representatives or delegates typically serving two-year terms (The White House, n.d.-b).

State judicial branches are usually led by a state supreme court. Like the Supreme Court at the federal level, state supreme courts do not conduct trials. Rather, their role is to hear appeals from lower-level state courts and correct errors made in those courts. State supreme court justices may be appointed by their governors or may be elected by the citizens of the state (The White House, n.d.-b). Whether state supreme court justices have term limits is determined by individual state constitutions. Some state constitutions allow for appellate courts that are geographically determined circuit courts, similar to the federal level.

In addition to state governments, there are local governments, which operate at two tiers:

- Counties, also known as boroughs (Alaska) or parishes (Louisiana), which may be further divided into entities called townships
- Municipalities, also known as cities or towns

Local governments can be structured in many different ways, as defined by their state constitutions, and are variable in size from small towns to cities the size of New York City (population 8 million), Los Angeles (population 3.7 million), and Chicago (population 2.6 million) (CityMayors, 2010; The White House, n.d.-b).

The Structure and Function of Executive Branch Agencies and Regulatory Boards

Executive branch agencies are created by federal, state, or municipal law and exist at all three levels. They are a formal part of the executive branch of government. Because they are created in law, their powers and duties are established in and granted by law. They report to and serve at the will of the executive branch of government.

Examples of federal cabinet-level departments were provided earlier. Examples of cabinet-level departments at the state level include departments of health, aging, administrative services, and developmental disabilities. At the local level, executive branch departments are often responsible for the regulation of sanitation and health issues, retail food safety, construction, waste disposal, health-code enforcement, and the reporting of communicable disease to state and federal authorities. Local health departments may also offer services such as free clinics, HIV/AIDS testing, tuberculosis clinics, and dental or immunization programs.

The heads of executive branch departments may be appointed by the commander in chief (the president of the US for federal departments and the governor for state departments). In the case of state regulatory agencies or boards, many of which are created to regulate a profession, the law generally calls for the creation of a board, which is appointed by the governor. Many regulatory agency laws specify that board members then elect a president from among themselves.

The primary purpose of regulatory agencies is to protect the public safety and welfare, and agencies are structured accordingly. While enforcing the law is ultimately the responsibility of the appointed board, it is the staff that conducts the day-to-day business specified in law and in rule. As such, executive branch regulatory agency board appointees generally hire an executive director, who in turn hires and manages a staff. Some of the work that a regulatory agency oversees may include investigative or compliance work.

State executive branch regulatory agencies must follow administrative procedures and guidelines, which are outlined in the state's Administrative Procedures Act (APA). The APA sets out rules regarding the conduct of state agencies and procedures agencies must follow to promulgate (write) rules.

The laws that create departments and agencies are general in nature and must be amplified for their daily operations to be carried out. To do this, the department or agency is given rulemaking authority in law. Rules may only amplify existing law; they may not supersede law or conflict with another department or agency's laws or rules. This process is described in detail in Chapter 5, "Policymaking Processes and Models." As an example, the state of Ohio's APA asserts that a new or revised rule:

- May not exceed the agency's statutory authority
- Does not conflict with an existing rule of that agency or any other state agency
- Does not conflict with legislative intent

The Ohio APA also requires that the rule-making agency complete an accurate rule summary and fiscal analysis and that the agency or board prepare an impact analysis if necessary.

Further, the APA in Ohio requires that a joint committee of the legislature review the rule to ensure these mandates are met (Joint Committee on Agency Rule Review – Ohio General Assembly, 2018). For example, a board of nursing, by rule, could expand APRN practice to specify requirements for APRNs prescribing opioids for acute pain but could not expand APRN practice to include the dispensing of drugs, which is part of the scope of practice covered in the Pharmacy Practice Act. A rule cannot exceed the original legislative intent; therefore, it cannot change or expand scope of practice.

Structurally, state executive branch departments and regulatory agencies are public agencies (as are federal departments and agencies) and are therefore subject to the following:

- **Open meeting laws:** These laws govern the ability of the public to access governmental meetings (Ballotpedia, n.d.-a), although public governmental bodies are normally permitted to enter into executive (closed) sessions for specific reasons—for example, to discuss disciplinary or personnel matters, obtain legal advice from their attorneys, or conduct contract negotiations (Loversidge, 2019).

- **State sunshine laws:** These laws similarly regulate public access to governmental records. These are known as *open records* or *public records* laws; they are also referred to as *FOIA* **laws** (FOIA is short for the federal Freedom of Information Act) (Ballotpedia, n.d.-b).

State boards—in particular, health professions boards, including boards of nursing—may be structured as independent boards or as part of an umbrella board. An independent board is single-purposed, whereas an umbrella board is part of a consolidated regulatory organization that shares staff and resources. There are advantages and disadvantages to either model (Benton, Brekken, Ridenour, & Thomas, 2016).

Summary

This chapter began by considering the balance of power provided by the three branches of government: legislative, executive, and judicial. It followed with an overview of the structure and function of each of the three branches, using the US federal government as the model. Details regarding the Senate, House of Representatives, committee structures, the Office of the President of the US, the cabinet, and the Supreme Court and lower courts were discussed. Following that, the chapter covered the general organization of state governments. Finally, the chapter described executive branch departments and agencies as well as regulatory boards, with a focus on their structure and function.

References

Acs, A. (2016). Which statute to implement? Strategic timing by regulatory agencies. *Journal of Public Administration Research and Theory, 26*(3), 493–506. doi:10.1093/jopart/muv018

Ballotpedia. (n.d.-a). State open meetings laws. Retrieved from https://ballotpedia.org/State_open_meetings_laws

Ballotpedia. (n.d.-b). State sunshine laws. Retrieved from https://ballotpedia.org/State_sunshine_laws

Ballotpedia. (n.d.-c). States with gubernatorial term limits. Retrieved from https://ballotpedia.org/States_with_gubernatorial_term_limits

Benton, D., Brekken, S. A., Ridenour, J., & Thomas, K. (2016). Comparing performance of umbrella and independent nursing boards: An initial review. *Journal of Nursing Regulation, 7*(3), 52–57. doi:10.1016/S2155-8256(16)32324-9

Budget House Committee. (2018). Basics of the current federal budget process. Retrieved from https://budget.house.gov/budget-digest/basics-current-federal-budget-process/

CityMayors. (2010). The largest US cities: Cities Ranked 1 to 100. Retrieved from http://www.citymayors.com/gratis/uscities_100.html

Committee on House Administration. (n.d.-a). Congressional member and staff organizations. Retrieved from https://cha.house.gov/member-services/congressional-memberstaff-organizations

Committee on House Administration. (n.d.-b). 115th Congress congressional member organizations. Retrieved from https://cha.house.gov/sites/republicans.cha.house.gov/files/documents/115CMOList%282.6.17%29.pdf

Cornell Law School. (n.d.). Executive power. Retrieved from https://www.law.cornell.edu/wex/executive_power

Federal Register. (n.d.). Executive orders. Retrieved from https://www.federalregister.gov/executive-orders

Gerrymandering. (n.d.). *Encyclopedia Brittanica.* Retrieved from https://www.britannica.com/topic/gerrymandering

GovTrack. (n.d.). District of Columbia. Retrieved from https://www.govtrack.us/congress/members/DC

Hakim, J. (2007). *A history of US: From colonies to country: 1735–1791.* Oxford, UK: Oxford University Press.

Heitshusen, V. (2017). Committee types and roles. Retrieved from https://www.senate.gov/CRSpubs/312b4df4-9797-41bf-b623-a8087cc91d74.pdf

The Heritage Guide to the Constitution. (2017). Reserved powers of the states. Retrieved from https://www.heritage.org/constitution/#!/amendments/10/essays/163/reserved-powers-of-the-states

Joint Committee on Agency Rule Review – Ohio General Assembly. (2018). Welcome to JCARR. Retrieved from http://www.jcarr.state.oh.us/home

Loversidge, J. M. (2019). Government response: Regulation. In J. A. Milstead & N. M. Short (Eds.), *Health policy & politics: A nurse's guide* (6th ed., pp. 57–86). Burlington, MA: Jones & Bartlett Learning.

National Conference of State Legislatures. (n.d.). The federal budget process. Retrieved from http://www.ncsl.org/research/fiscal-policy/federal-budget-process.aspx

Rundquist, P. S. (n.d.). Resident commissioner from Puerto Rico: Prepared for members and committees of Congress. Retrieved from http://congressionalresearch.com/RL31856/document.php?study=Resident+Commissioner+from+Puerto+Rico

Supreme Court of the US. (n.d.-a). The court and constitutional interpretation. Retrieved from https://www.supremecourt.gov/about/constitutional.aspx

Supreme Court of the US. (n.d.-b). FAQs – general information. Retrieved from https://www.supremecourt.gov/about/faq_general.aspx

US Courts. (n.d.-a). About the Supreme Court. Retrieved from http://www.uscourts.gov/about-federal-courts/educational-resources/about-educational-outreach/activity-resources/about

US Courts. (n.d.-b). Court role and structure. Retrieved from http://www.uscourts.gov/about-federal-courts/court-role-and-structure

US House of Representatives. (n.d.-a). Committees. Retrieved from https://www.house.gov/committees

US House of Representatives. (n.d.-b). Directory of representatives. Retrieved from https://www.house.gov/representatives

US House of Representatives. (n.d.-c). Leadership. Retrieved from https://www.house.gov/leadership

US House of Representatives. (n.d.-d). Officers and organizations of the House. Retrieved from https://www.house.gov/the-house-explained/officers-and-organizations

US House of Representatives: History, Art & Archives. (n.d.-a). Constitutional qualifications. Retrieved from http://history.house.gov/Institution/Origins-Development/Constitutional-Qualifications/

US House of Representatives: History, Art & Archives. (n.d.-b). Meet the people of the people's house. Retrieved from http://history.house.gov/People/

US House of Representatives Office of the Historian. (n.d.). Speaker of the house. Retrieved from: https://history.house.gov/Institution/Origins-Development/Speaker-of-the-House/

US Senate. (n.d.-a). About the Senate committee system. Retrieved from https://www.senate.gov/general/common/generic/about_committees.htm

US Senate. (n.d.-b). Committees. Retrieved from https://www.senate.gov/committees/index.htm

US Senate. (n.d.-c). Glossary term: Override of a veto. Retrieved from https://www.senate.gov/reference/glossary_term/override_of_a_veto.htm

US Senate. (n.d.-d). Leadership & officers. Retrieved from http://www.senate.gov/senators/leadership.htm

US Senate. (n.d.-e). Officers & staff. Retrieved from https://www.senate.gov/pagelayout/reference/two_column_table/Officers_and_Staff.htm

US Senate. (n.d.-f). Origins and development. Retrieved from https://www.senate.gov/artandhistory/history/common/briefing/Origins_Development.htm

US Senate. (n.d.-g). Secretary of the Senate. Retrieved from https://www.senate.gov/reference/office/secretary_of_senate.htm

US Senate. (n.d.-h). Senate committees. Retrieved from https://www.senate.gov/artandhistory/history/common/briefing/Committees.htm#2

US Senate. (n.d.-i). Senators. Retrieved from https://www.senate.gov/reference/reference_index_subjects/Senators_vrd.htm

USA.gov. (2018). Branches of the U.S. government. Retrieved from https://www.usa.gov/branches-of-government

UShistory.org. (2018). How judges and justices are chosen. Retrieved from http://www.ushistory.org/gov/9d.asp

USLegal.com. (2016). US courts of appeals. Retrieved from https://system.uslegal.com/us-courts-of-appeals/

Warrington, G. S. (2018). Quantifying gerrymandering using the vote distribution. *Election Law Journal, 17*(1), 39–57. doi:10.1089/elj.2017.0447

The White House. (n.d.-a). Our government: The executive branch. Retrieved from https://www.whitehouse.gov/about-the-white-house/the-executive-branch/

The White House. (n.d.-b). Our government: State & local government. Retrieved from https://www.whitehouse.gov/about-the-white-house/state-local-government/

"The political process does not end on Election Day . . . stay involved in the process by continuing to pay attention to the conversation and holding . . . leaders accountable for the decisions they make."

–Patrick Murphy

5

POLICYMAKING PROCESSES AND MODELS

–JACQUELINE M. LOVERSIDGE, PHD, RNC-AWHC

KEY CONTENT IN THIS CHAPTER

- How a bill becomes a law
- How regulations are made
- Policy process frameworks and models
- Partisan politics, the importance of cost, stakeholder influence, and expert opinion

How a Bill Becomes a Law

If you grew up during the 1970s, you probably remember watching *School-house Rock*, a series of short educational cartoons that explained the ins and outs of topics like grammar, math, and more. Among the most famous of these was one called "I'm Just a Bill," which offered a simplified but accurate portrayal of how a bill becomes a law (Disney Educational Productions, 2011). Indeed, this short cartoon became such a classic, it appears on GovTrack, a website designed to help Americans participate in their government, as an introduction to the process.

In reality, the process of lawmaking is arduous, complex, and virtually never linear. In the US Congress, very few bills that are introduced ever become law. For example, in the 114th congressional session, which began in January 2015 and ended in January 2017, only 3% of the bills introduced were enacted into law, comprising just 329 laws. The 113th Congress passed even fewer laws (296 laws), and the 112th Congress passed fewer still (284 laws) (GovTrack, 2018b). States have a similar success rate (or lack thereof).

As noted, in the United States, laws are passed by the legislative branch of the government. The US Congress passes laws at the federal level, while state legislative bodies pass laws at the state level. (The structure and function of these bodies are described in Chapter 4, "Government Structures and Functions That Drive Process.")

At the federal level, any individual, group, or legislator might identify an idea for a bill. From the time someone conceives of an idea for a new bill or a revision to an existing bill and the time that bill is signed into law, the bill must undergo a number of steps (GovTrack, 2018a; USA.gov, 2018):

1. Someone has an idea for a new or revised law.

2. A bill is introduced and referred to committee.

3. The bill goes to committee for consideration.

4. The bill is added to the chamber's calendar for consideration.

5. The House or Senate debates and votes on the bill (depending on which chamber the bill started in).

6. The other chamber votes on the bill.

7. Differences are resolved.

8. The president approves or vetoes the bill.

9. The law is assigned a number and incorporated into the US Code.

Of course, politics and a host of process details add complications and time to each of these steps. Figure 5.1 shows a simplified visual representation of how a bill becomes a law. What's important to note is that there are numerous points during this process at which evidence can be used to affect the outcome. (There are other forms of legislation such as resolutions, but bills are the most common and will be discussed here.)

> State legislatures follow many of the same steps and processes.

Step 1: Someone Has an Idea for a New or Revised Law

The idea for a new law or for a revision of an existing law can come from any source. One common source for ideas is constituents. Constituents often talk to their representatives in Congress about specific problems in their district that may have an impact on citizens across the country. If the problem is widespread enough to warrant the attention of the federal government, their congressional representatives may decide the issue is one worth addressing through legislation.

Another source of ideas for bills is professional or trade organizations. Special interest organizations often press congressional representatives to take up their causes in legislation. Organizations with *political action committees* (PACs) that make campaign donations frequently find favor with their legislators— the greater the donation, the greater the influence. For example, in 2017, the American Nurses Association spent $1,563,021 on lobbying (Center for Responsive Politics [CRP], n.d.-b). By comparison, the American Medical Association spent $21,525,000 on lobbying (CRP, n.d.-a), and the healthcare industry at large, without considering organized nursing or medicine, spent $561,231,163 (CRP, n.d.-c).

Finally, legislators frequently identify changes in law they would like to effect based on their own experience. If passed, these laws are often considered part of their congressional legacy.

HOW DOES A BILL BECOME A LAW?

① EVERY LAW STARTS WITH AN IDEA

That idea can come from anyone, even you! Contact your elected officials to share your idea. If they want to try to make it a law, they will write a bill.

② THE BILL IS INTRODUCED

A bill can start in either house of Congress when it's introduced by its primary sponsor, a Senator or a Representative. In the House of Representatives, bills are placed in a wooden box called "the hopper."

③ THE BILL GOES TO COMMITTEE

Representatives or Senators meet in a small group to research, talk about, and make changes to the bill. They vote to accept or reject the bill and its changes before sending it to:

the House or Senate floor for debate or to a subcommittee for further research.

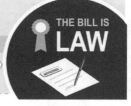

Here, the bill is assigned a legislative number before the Speaker of the House sends it to a committee.

④ CONGRESS DEBATES AND VOTES

Members of the House or Senate can now debate the bill and propose changes or amendments before voting. If the majority vote for and pass the bill, it moves to the other house to go through a similar process of committees, debate, and voting. Both houses have to agree on the same version of the final bill before it goes to the President.

DID YOU KNOW?

The House uses an electronic voting system while the Senate typically votes by voice, saying "yay" or "nay."

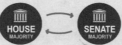

HOUSE MAJORITY ⟷ SENATE MAJORITY

⑤ PRESIDENTIAL ACTION

When the bill reaches the President, he or she can:

✓ **APPROVE and PASS**
The President signs and approves the bill. The bill is law.

THE BILL IS **LAW**

The President can also:

Veto
The President rejects the bill and returns it to Congress with the reasons for the veto. Congress can override the veto with 2/3 vote of those present in both the House and the Senate and the bill will become law.

Choose no action
The President can decide to do nothing. If Congress is in session, after 10 days of no answer from the President, the bill then automatically becomes law.

Pocket veto
If Congress adjourns (goes out of session) within the 10 day period after giving the President the bill, the President can choose not to sign it and the bill will not become law.

Brought to you by usa gov

FIGURE 5.1 How does a bill become a law?
(Image courtesy of USA.gov)

After an idea is generated, it must be written down in bill form. Anyone can draft the ideas included in a bill—indeed, early drafts of bill language often come from stakeholders (Magleby, Monroe, & Robinson, 2018)—but a member of Congress or his or her legislative aides must draft the bill according to strict guidelines specific to the House (Office of the Legislative Counsel: US House of Representatives, n.d.) or Senate (Office of the Legislative Counsel: US Senate, n.d.). During this process, negotiations ensue between the stakeholder interest groups and the potential sponsor, resulting in many drafts and comments on those drafts. Because this process is complicated and often time-consuming, the idea step and the drafting step are considered to be integrated.

Step 2: A Bill Is Introduced and Referred to Committee

After a bill is drafted, it is introduced into either the House or the Senate, depending on who serves as the primary legislative sponsor of the bill. Only chamber members introduce bills, although a member may introduce legislation at the president's request.

It is advantageous for a bill to have bipartisan primary co-sponsorship. This occurs when two or more primary sponsors belonging to opposing political parties find sufficient common ground to support the same issue (Rambur, 2017). To achieve this, the bill's initial sponsor circulates the bill to other members of the chamber and requests that their colleagues sign on as co-sponsors to demonstrate support.

In the House, the bill is introduced when it is dropped into what's called the *Hopper*—a wooden box on the House floor. In the Senate, the bill is submitted to Senate clerks on the floor. Bills introduced in the House contain the letters *HR* in their name, while the names of bills introduced in the Senate contain an *S*. Bills are also given a number, which is the next number available, in sequence, during that two-year congressional session (Congress.gov, n.d.-d).

A commonly employed strategy is to introduce *companion bills*. These are bills that are identical and introduced simultaneously in both the Senate and the House. Lawmakers may use this strategy to promote simultaneous consideration. This method enables proponents of a particular piece of legislation to take advantage of the process in the chamber in which it is getting the most traction to enable its swift passage.

After a bill is introduced, it is referred to committee. In the House, the speaker refers bills to committee with involvement from a nonpartisan parliamentarian advisor. The chamber's standing rules guide referral to all committees that have jurisdiction over any provisions contained in the bill, although most bills are heard in only one committee. If multiple committees are involved, one will likely take the lead. The Senate generally follows a similar process, but some bills may go directly to the Senate floor for consideration following a series of prescribed procedural steps (Congress.gov, n.d.-d).

Step 3: The Bill Goes to Committee for Consideration

Bills that are referred to committee go through three formal committee actions:

1. **A hearing:** A hearing is a public forum during which committee members may hear from interested parties—proponents and opponents—about the bill's strengths and weaknesses. Industry organization representatives, leaders from executive branch agencies, and interested citizens may testify. Witness testimony is provided in writing for the record, but shorter oral statements may also be offered; this provides committee members an opportunity to ask questions.

   > Because committees often receive more bills than they are able to pursue to fruition, some bills never reach the hearing stage. The committee chair decides which bills do and don't get heard.

2. **Markup:** The committee chair determines which version of the bill will be considered by the committee for markup. This is when amendments or substitutions may be made. (These are common; rarely does a bill move through both houses without some change.) Markup only occurs if there is a high degree of confidence that the bill will be successfully voted out of committee. During markup, both House and Senate committees may also establish subcommittees in which elements of a bill can be considered in greater detail. Subcommittees must report back to the full parent committee before the bill can be reported out to the full chamber (Congress.gov, n.d.-b).

3. **Reporting:** After the hearing and markup phases, the committee reports the bill to the full chamber by majority vote. The report is an official publication in which the congressional committee makes a recommendation to the whole House or Senate. It may include committee hearing findings, deliberation outcomes, discussion of legislative intent, a brief history of the bill, and a comparison between the proposed law text and current law. Most reports make recommendations for passage of the piece of legislation that has been considered by the committee during hearings and in private session (LexisNexis, 2007).

Bills are particularly at risk of failure during a lame duck session, when Congress is about to adjourn at the end of a term. This occurs during even-numbered years following November elections, when it becomes clear that some lawmakers will not be returning for the next congressional session because they have lost an election, are term-limited, or are retiring (Egan, 2004). During a lame duck session, to move legislation through the process, lame duck politicians often resort to making deals to tack legislation onto unrelated bills or amendments—like hanging ornaments on a holiday tree. These are colloquially known as *Christmas tree bills.*

Step 4: The Bill Is Added to the Chamber's Calendar for Consideration

After a bill has been reported out by committee, it is placed on the chamber's calendar and considered for floor action. Not all bills placed on the calendar will reach the floor during the two-year congressional session, however. In the House, majority party leadership, with consultation from committee leaders, generally decides which bills the full chamber will consider. Or, House leadership may ask the Rules Committee to bring a bill to the floor if they anticipate that the bill will require more detailed consideration.

The Senate process is somewhat different. The Senate can agree to a motion to proceed, which allows a bill to be heard on the floor, after debate of the motion and agreement by majority vote. The Senate majority leader may also ask for unanimous consent that the Senate agree to hear a bill. The bill may then be considered immediately if there is no objection. If a senator objects—in which case he or she is said to have placed a *hold* on the bill—the leader is unlikely to request unanimous consent (Congress.gov, n.d.-a).

After a bill has been scheduled, the House or Senate can debate and vote on the bill according to their unique procedures.

Step 5: The House Debates and Votes on the Bill

The House has its own unique set of rules and procedures for considering a bill. Most often, it uses a procedure called *suspension of the rules.* This procedure limits debate to 40 minutes and prohibits members from offering amendments on the floor. A bill passing under these rules requires a two-thirds vote; only bills with supermajority support in the House will pass. Bills not considered under suspension of the rules are considered on a case-by-case basis through the adoption of a simple House resolution, or special rule, reported by the House Rules Committee.

House procedures require that any amendments must meet the standard of germaneness. That is, they must be on subject with the bill's content to be considered. When amendments meet this requirement, the House considers the bill for the purpose of voting on amendments in a procedural setting called the *Committee of the Whole*. Once that is done, the Committee of the Whole reports to the full House with recommended amendments and the allowance of amendments by the minority party. Then electronic vote by the full House may occur (Congress.gov, n.d.-c).

At times, bills may be held up in committee. If this happens to a bill that has been referred to committee for 30 or more legislative days, any member of the House may file a motion with the clerk of the House to discharge the committee from further consideration of the bill or resolution and bring the bill to the floor for consideration. This is called a *discharge petition*. A majority of the House—218 members—must sign the discharge petition within a certain time frame for the bill to be considered (US House of Representatives Committee on Rules Majority Office, n.d.).

Step 6: The Senate Debates and Votes on the Bill

The Senate rules of conduct are considerably different from those in the House. The Senate must agree to consider a bill on the floor by either agreeing to a unanimous consent request or by voting to adopt a motion to proceed to the bill. After agreement to consider the bill has been reached, senators may debate and propose amendments. There is no limit on the amount of time senators have to debate amendments or the bill itself.

One unique feature of the Senate's process is the filibuster. A *filibuster* is an extended debate with the intent to delay or prevent a final vote. A filibuster can threaten passage on amendments, bills, or motions. However, the Senate cloture rule (Senate Rule XXII) allows a supermajority to limit both debate and amendments that may be offered. This rule allows the Senate to stop a filibuster by limiting consideration of a pending matter to 30 additional hours. Cloture requires a vote of three-fifths of the full Senate, which normally constitutes 60 votes (US Senate, n.d.).

A more effective means of limiting debate and amendments is the *unanimous consent agreement,* which can be customized to a specific bill. This is essentially a contract upon which all senators agree to allow for effective process and procedural rights of members.

Much voting in the Senate is by voice vote, although at times a recorded roll-call vote is required or requested. The Senate does not have an electronic voting system, as does the House (Congress.gov, n.d.-g). Electronic voting was introduced in the House in 1973 (US House of Representatives: History, Art & Archives, n.d.).

Step 7: Differences Are Resolved

Before a bill can be presented to the president for signature, it must be agreed to by both chambers. After a bill passes one chamber—whether the House or the Senate—it is engrossed, or prepared in official form, and then sent to the other chamber. The second chamber might agree to the bill as it has been passed in the first chamber, or it might decide to amend the bill or offer a different version of it for consideration. If the second chamber passes the bill in an amended or alternative form, it must send the bill back to the first chamber for concurrence. (That is, the first chamber must concur with the changes.) The first chamber may then offer a counterproposal. This process, called an *amendment exchange,* could go on between the chambers indefinitely, until the congressional session ends. Eventually, the bill must be agreed to before it can move on to the president.

An alternative for resolving differences between the House and Senate is for the bill to go through conference committee. This is a temporary committee comprised of members of both the House and the Senate who attempt to reach a compromise bill. If a compromise bill is reached in conference committee, its report is considered first in one chamber, then the other. Both chambers must agree to the conference report without changes for the bill to move on to the president (Congress.gov, n.d.-f).

Step 8: The President Approves or Vetoes the Bill

After both the House and the Senate have agreed to the bill, it is *enrolled,* which means it is prepared in final form and sent to the White House for the president's signature. The president has 10 days (excluding Sundays) to either sign or veto the bill. If the president signs the bill during that period, it becomes law. If the president vetoes the bill, it is returned to the original chamber, which may attempt to override the veto by a two-thirds vote. If override is successful in the original chamber, the other chamber also has the option to vote to override the veto—again, requiring a two-thirds vote. A presidential veto can be overridden only if both chambers garner adequate votes, which is rare (Congress.gov, n.d.-f). If the president fails to sign or veto the bill, the bill becomes law without the president's signature, except under certain circumstances when Congress has adjourned (Congress.gov, n.d.-e). This is called a *pocket veto*.

Step 9: The Law Is Assigned a Number and Incorporated Into the US Code

After a bill is enacted, the Office of the Federal Register at the National Archives assigns the bill a public law number. Then the law is published in the next edition of the *United Statutes at Large* (Congress.gov, n.d.-f), which is the permanent collection of laws and resolutions enacted during each congressional session. These are archived and available electronically back to the first session of the 82nd Congress in 1951 (US Government Publishing Office, n.d.).

How Regulations Are Made

Laws establish legislative intent but usually require detail before they can be implemented. This detail is conveyed in the form of regulations (also referred to as rules and administrative code). Put a different way, laws give direction to the administrative agency that will write, or promulgate, related regulations.

Regulations are not synonymous with law. However, because they are adopted under statutory authority, they have the force and effect of law (Regulations, n.d.) and are essential to a law's implementation. As with lawmaking, rulemaking is a public process, although it is significantly less complicated and involves only a single governmental agency.

Governmental agencies at all levels operate to enforce regulations. A governmental agency gets its authority to issue regulations from the laws enacted by

Congress or, at the state level, from laws enacted by the state legislature. In the case of federal law, federal departments generate federal regulations. State departments have much the same role: to generate state regulations. On occasion, the president may delegate presidential authority to an agency to issue rules.

Typically, when Congress or a state legislature creates an agency, it also grants that agency general authority to issue rules. The agency's rulemaking authority must not exceed its statutory authority or it risks violating the US Constitution or state constitution (depending on whether the agency is a federal or state agency).

Once each year, in the fall, federal agencies are required to publish a regulatory plan. Twice a year, in the spring and fall, they must publish an agenda of regulatory and deregulatory actions. Together, these two documents are referred to as the *unified agenda*. The unified agenda is a public document that is posted on RegInfo.gov and Regulations.gov. The Government Printing Office (GPO) also publishes a version in the *Federal Register*.

Federal rulemaking requirements are described in the Administrative Procedures Act of 1946 (Carey, 2013). Roughly speaking, the rulemaking process is as follows (see Figure 5.2), although not all rules must follow all the steps seen in the figure:

1. The need for a rule becomes clear.

2. The agency rule is drafted and reviewed.

3. The proposed rule is rolled out to the public.

4. The agency reviews input and costs and finalizes the rule.

5. The agency publishes the final rule.

> Rulemaking is another point at which evidence can be used to drive outcomes favorable to stakeholders.

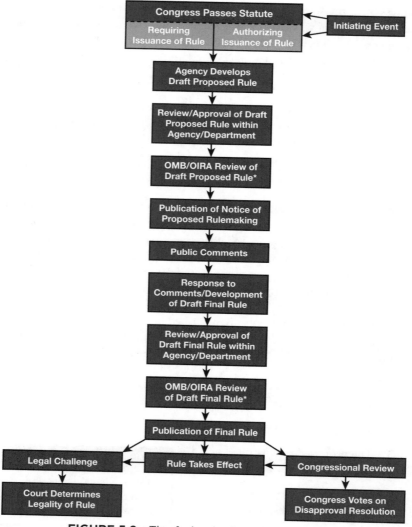

FIGURE 5.2   The federal rulemaking process.
(Image courtesy of the Congressional Research Service)

The Office of Management and Budget (OBM) Office of Information and Regulatory Affairs (OIRA) reviews only significant rules and does not review any rules submitted by independent regulatory agencies. Reproduced from Carey, 2013.

Step 1: The Need for a Rule Becomes Clear

Agencies make rules when a law that changes the agency's charge on a certain subject is passed or when the agency reviews its area of legal responsibility and identifies a policy priority, issue, or need for clarification that would be served by rulemaking (Office of the Federal Register, 2011). For example, Congress could pass a new statute that requires that rules be written to amplify a rule, or the statute might directly authorize the issuance of a rule. Regardless, some initiating event begins the process.

Step 2: The Agency Rule Is Drafted and Reviewed

Generally speaking, the rule-drafting process begins when regulatory agency staff familiar with the regulations draft the proposed rule. The draft is reviewed and approved within the department and is then sent to the Office of Management and Budget (OMB) for review of budgetary considerations or to other federal departments as necessary.

When these initial steps are completed, the federal agency must publish a document called an *advance notice of proposed rulemaking* in the *Federal Register*. This is done so that any individuals or groups who wish to provide public comment on the rule as it is being developed may do so.

Some agencies develop proposed rules through a process of negotiated rule-making with the public—particularly professional or trade organizations. When this process is successful, an agency may use the ideas from this negotiation as the basis for the proposed rule (Office of the Federal Register, 2011). States follow a similar public process; requirements for public notice and other procedures are found in state administrative procedures acts.

Step 3: The Proposed Rule Is Rolled Out to the Public

After an agency drafts a rule, it files a *notice of proposed rulemaking* (NPRM). This official document explains the rule's purpose to the public. All proposed federal rules are published in the *Federal Register* and include a public comment period, which generally ranges from 30 to 60 days, although up to 180 days may be permitted for more complex rules. The agency may or may not consider comments filed following the end of the comment period (Office of the Federal Register, 2011).

If agencies find additional comment is needed, they may reopen the comment period. The agency may also hold public hearings. Some agencies are required to hold public rulemaking hearings; others are not. Most agencies prefer electronically submitted comments so they are easily available to the public. Instructions for providing comment are found in the *Federal Register* on the Regulations.gov Help pages (Office of the Federal Register, 2011).

Step 4: The Agency Reviews Input and Costs and Finalizes the Rule

After the comment period is over, the agency compiles public comments, evaluates proponent and opponent commentary, and considers all information in context. The agency is required to base its rationale and conclusions for the rulemaking record on commentary provided by the public. It is also required to justify its rationale and conclusions on relevant science, expert opinion, and other facts gathered during the pre-rule and proposed-rule stages (Office of the Federal Register, 2011). States may not have such rulemaking requirements.

After the agency has concluded that the proposed rule is a rational solution to an identified problem or will help achieve an identified goal, it must also consider cost-effectiveness. New considerations may require changes in the rule as drafted at that point. If major changes are required, a supplemental proposed rule is published; if the changes are minor, the agency may proceed with drafting of a final rule. The agency conducts a final intradepartmental review and approval of the draft final rule before it is sent on for final review.

Before the rule is published in the *Federal Register*, the president and the Office of Information and Regulatory Affairs (OIRA) and the OMB review the draft proposed rules. During this process, final estimated costs and benefits are analyzed, and any alternative solutions suggested in public comments may be considered. During this time agencies may also consult with other agencies with which they share responsibility for items addressed by the rule. In some cases, interagency review is mandatory (Office of the Federal Register, 2011).

Step 5: The Agency Publishes the Final Rule

After all reviews are complete, the final rule is published, and the rule takes effect. Final rules are structured with a preamble, summary, effective date, and supplementary information. Afterward, they are published in the *Federal Register*.

In this documentation, agencies must transparently state the basis and purpose of the rule and describe the goals or problems addressed with the rule and the evidence upon which the agency relied to draft the rule. Any major public criticisms of the rule must be addressed and, if applicable, an explanation as to why the agency chose not to respond to public critique with an alternative included. Finally, the agency must indicate what section(s) of law grant it the authority to issue the rule. Rules generally go into effect 30 days after publication in the *Federal Register*, with exceptions for "good cause" (Office of the Federal Register, 2011).

Changes to the Code of Federal Regulations (CFR) must be published by the agency in the final rule. When they become effective, rules are also found in the Electronic Code of Federal Regulations (e-CFR) database (https://www.ecfr.gov/). The e-CFR is not the official publication but is considered reputable and authoritative and is compiled by the Office of the Federal Register and GPO. More detailed information about each of these steps can be found at the Office of the Federal Register (2011).

State Rulemaking Processes

Although the rulemaking processes followed by state governments may differ in their details, overall, they are similar to the federal process. The rule in its final form is filed with the appropriate state department. State rules normally go through a joint legislative committee evaluation process much like the presidential/OIRA process and must meet the following standards:

- They must be written based on the legislative authority in the agency's statute.
- They must not conflict with other agencies' laws or rules.

An effective date is established, per the state administrative code, based on the date of final filing (Loversidge, 2019).

Policy Process Frameworks and Models

Familiarity with some of the most commonly used policymaking frameworks and models will enable you to recognize political and other actions and structures that can facilitate or hinder the process of policymaking and provide insight into points at which evidence can provide the greatest leverage during the lawmaking or rulemaking processes. These frameworks and models include the following:

- Kingdon's streams model
- Sabatier's Advocacy Coalition Framework
- The CDC policy analytical framework
- Force-field analysis

Kingdon's Streams Model

John Kingdon's streams model was introduced in 1984, and its use continues today. Indeed, it has been applied in many studies of policy across the globe (Rawat & Morris, 2016).

Kingdon (1995) lays the foundation for the model by suggesting that two factors make government actors notice an idea and then act on that idea: participants and processes. Participants are individuals who may be visible and influential in agenda setting, such as the president or members of Congress, or less visible, such as governmental staff or bureaucrats. The work of governmental staff and bureaucrats is to suggest policy alternatives rather than set the agenda (Kingdon, 1995; Rawat & Morris, 2016). However, the work of governmental staff and bureaucrats can have significant influence on the policy agenda.

As for processes, Kingdon (1995) identifies three essential types in policy formulation, called *streams*. These are as follows:

- **The problem stream:** In Kingdon's (1995) model, the problem stream begins to flow when societal attention is directed to a problem amenable to a policy solution. This attention can result from an indicator such as the recognition of the data pattern emerging from the opioid crisis. It can also result from a one-time crisis—for example, a bridge collapse necessitating the institution of a government program of bridge inspection and repair. Finally, it can result from a symbol that represents a public problem. This was the case with the photographs of children separated from immigrant parents crossing the border from Mexico into the US in 2018. The stories of desperate parents unable to gain access to information about their children's location, and viral images of some lawmakers seeking to unite them, became symbolic of the time and associated policy problem.

- **The policy stream:** The policy stream refers to the many potential policy solutions that arise from the various communities of policy-makers, special interest and lobbying groups, and government experts and bureaucrats. Kingdon calls this a "policy primeval soup" (1995, p. 117) because of the variety of stakeholders involved, the potential complexity of issues, and the abundance of lively debate that can occur in this policy stream.

- **The politics stream:** The politics stream is independent of the other two streams. It is formed from the communities of interests who have a stake in the problem and in its method of solution. As this stream flows, ideas are formed, proposals are generated, and policy drafts are written and redrafted. If all goes well, collaborative efforts aim toward the target—the policy window. Public mood, special interest group and campaign group pressure, and partisan politics all have an effect on this stream, as does the overall policy agenda (Howlett, Mc-Connell, & Perl, 2015; Kingdon, 1995).

If and when the problem, policy, and politics streams converge, the result is public policy. Kingdon refers to this convergence as the *joining of streams* or the *policy window*. Forces such as partisan politics, election results, and national interest may converge to realign the political agenda and drive a particular policy problem to the top, therefore opening the policy window and allowing the joined problem, policy, and politics streams to pass through into policy (Howlett, McConnell, & Perl, 2015; Kingdon, 1995; Rawat & Morris, 2016). Many graphic interpretations and applications of this model exist; Figure 5.3 shows our interpretation of the model.

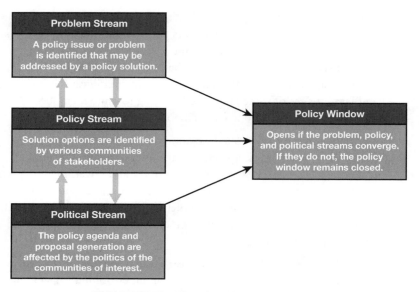

FIGURE 5.3   Kingdon's streams model.

Sabatier's Advocacy Coalition Framework

Sabatier (1988) and colleagues (Weible et al., 2011; Weible, Sabatier, & McQueen, 2009) developed and studied the use of the Advocacy Coalition Framework (ACF). The ACF describes and explains the complex policymaking environment, which is distinguished by several factors and attributes:

- Multiple actors and levels of government are involved.

- It is capable of decision-making, in spite of high levels of ambiguity and uncertainty.

- It accepts that the process of turning decisions into outcomes typically takes years.

- It suggests that policy processes differ according to the issues they address; some are intensely political and subject to dispute by various actors and stakeholders, while others are more technical and processed by policy specialists (for example, governmental agency staff) in less public venues.

The ACF relies on several key terms and concepts. These include the following:

- **Beliefs:** Individuals engage in politics to translate their beliefs into actions. According to Sabatier et al., the three main types of beliefs are as follows:
    - **Core:** Core beliefs are fundamental and unlikely to change. An example of a core belief is one's religion.
    - **Policy core:** Policy core beliefs are more specific. They are also unlikely to change. Examples of policy core beliefs include ideas on the balance between government and healthcare spending controls.
    - **Secondary aspects:** These relate to policy implementation. These are more likely to change as learning about policy aspects occurs.
- **Advocacy coalition:** This term refers to individuals from a variety of positions, including government officials, interest group leaders, citizens, or researchers, who share beliefs and coordinate their activities over time to achieve a policy goal.
- **Policy learning:** This describes a political process during which coalitions selectively interpret information and use it to leverage power.
- **Subsystems:** Coalitions subsystems are issue-specific networks that may compete with each other for dominance in policymaking.
- **Policy broker and sovereign:** Subsystems consist of actors who are in a position to mediate between coalitions and are authorized to make decisions on behalf of their coalition. Policymakers may be members of coalitions and serve in these roles.
- **Enlightenment:** This describes the change of a core belief—generally thought to be unchangeable—which may occur over the course of decades.

The ACF was originally developed to explain policymaking in the US. Over the years, the ACF has become a foundational framework for guiding inquiry by policy researchers. In that time, it has addressed several criticisms. One of these criticisms relates to its applicability to subsystems outside the US. In answer, dozens of researchers have applied the framework in a variety of international contexts, establishing its usefulness as a framework to guide and understand policymaking around the world (Weible et al., 2011).

The CDC Policy Analytical Framework

The Centers for Disease Control and Prevention (CDC, 2013) developed a policy analytical framework as "a guide for identifying, analyzing, and prioritizing policies that can improve health" (p. 3). The analytical framework describes domains I, II, and III of the CDC's overall policy process. These are as follows:

I. Problem Identification

II. Policy Analysis

III. Strategy and Policy Development

> The other two domains are IV, Policy Enactment, and V, Policy Implementation.

The policy analytical framework is a four-step model. The key steps are as follows (see Figure 5.4):

1. **Identify the problem or issue:** This step involves clearly identifying the problem or issue to be addressed and synthesizing data that characterizes the problem or issue. This includes the level of burden, frequency, severity, and scope.

2. **Identify an appropriate policy solution:** This step involves identifying policy options by following a process that includes reviewing the evidence, surveying best practices, and conducting an environmental scan to understand what is being done about the problem in other jurisdictions.

3. **Identify and describe policy options:** Each identified policy option must be clearly described as to process and structure. Key criteria and associated questions make necessary details transparent. For example:

   - Which policy lever is required (legislative, administrative, or regulatory)?
   - Which level of government will implement the policy?
   - What are the policy objectives?
   - What is the legal landscape (court rulings, constitutionality, and so on)?
   - What is the historical context?
   - What is the value of a particular policy option, or its return on investment (ROI)?

- What are potential short-, intermediate-, and long-term out-comes of the policy?

- What are possible unintended positive and negative conse-quences of the policy?

4. **Develop a strategy for furthering the adoption of a policy solution:** Use the answers to the questions in step 3 to rate policy options and determine the most rational approach.

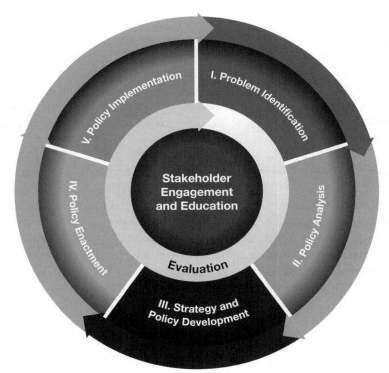

FIGURE 5.4 The CDC policy analytical framework model. *(Image courtesy of Centers for Disease Control and Prevention, Office of the Associate Director for Policy, 2015)*

Force-Field Analysis

Force-field analysis is a construction of social psychology and science. It is often attributed to Kurt Lewin's field theory (1939) but is in fact a later adaptation of Lewin's original work (Burnes & Cook, 2013).

Lewin's concept of planned change has provided useful tools for understanding, managing, and driving change. His original concept of planned change, which included field theory, was complex. He contributed four distinct ideas as a part of the concept of change: field theory, group dynamics, action research, and the three-step model of change. This last idea, the change model, involves unfreezing behavior from the status quo, implementing change, and refreezing, or stabilizing, in the new situation (Swanson & Creed, 2014). Lewin used field theory to explain an individual's behavior and behavior change relative to psychological forces in that person's life space and to explain how change arose from changes in those psychological forces.

As field theory was adapted for use in organizations and other settings, force-field analysis was developed (Burnes & Cook, 2013). Force-field analysis is helpful for analyzing causal relationships in a drive toward a particular change. In this context, the causal relationships are opposing; on one side are forces pressing for a policy change, and on the other are forces of resistance against that policy change. These forces are known as *enablers* and *constraints* in the force field (Swanson & Creed, 2014).

An example can be found in organizational policy change. In an academic medical center, nursing staff and leadership identified that several different policies guiding the care of patients with hyperglycemia had been approved for use. Policies were evidence-based but were located in different areas of the intranet and focused on different patient populations. For providers in a particular specialty area whose patients were especially prone to hyperglycemia, this presented problems because appropriate care delivery could be delayed or incomplete due to the difficulty in accessing the most relevant policy. APRN leads, with the support of nursing and physician leadership, followed organizational processes to: 1) consolidate the existing evidence-based guidelines; 2) enhance policy accessibility on the intranet; and 3) plan education and training regarding the changes for the end-user staff (Cordell, 2019).

In this example, enablers, or driving forces, included provider staff; among these were prescribing physicians and APRNs. Additionally, nursing and medical leadership fully supported this change, as did the RNs who carry out prescribers' orders. All are equally invested in the patient's care, and the expected outcome of this policy change is more efficient care of the patient at risk for hyperglycemia, and improved outcomes for that specialty population. Constraining forces may seem minimal because they were related to organizational structure; however, they were not insignificant. Teamwork on the part of the leadership and stakeholders overcame the constraining forces, and the policy change is expected to yield significant outcomes (see Table 5.1).

TABLE 5.1 Force-Field Analysis of an Organizational Policy Change Process

Enabling Forces	Tension Between Enabling and Constraining Forces	Constraining Forces
Provider staff, including prescribing physicians and APRNs, notice difficulty accessing multiple hyperglycemia policies located in various areas of organizational intranet		The organization's intranet does not accommodate easy access from multiple specialty areas of a complex organization
Provider staff (prescribing physicians and APRNs), implementing staff (RNs), and nursing and medical leadership united in their desire to improve hyperglycemia policy usability and accessibility		In a large organization, processes for policy change are in place and must be followed logically and sequentially
Full support for specialty area policy consolidation, education, and training, and organizational support for intranet posting		No equivalent constraining/resisting force

Swanson and Creed (2014) proposed an inverse principle based on Lewin's description of a paradoxical effect that, to reach a goal, it may at times be necessary to begin by moving in an opposite direction. With this in mind, enabling forces may be perceived as either a complement to achieving a goal or as a replacement for a performance. Conversely, constraining forces might be perceived as a barrier to the goal or as a motivator for change.

Partisan Politics, the Importance of Cost, Stakeholder Influence, and Expert Opinion

A discussion of the processes involved in policymaking must address the ways in which partisan politics, the importance of cost, the actions of stakeholders and other actors, and the opinions of experts contribute to the policymaking process. It is important to be aware that these influences are constantly at work; what is difficult is to appreciate that they are constantly in flux, hard to assess, and challenging to manage.

Partisan Politics

You've already learned in Chapter 4 about the roles of the president or governor, Senate leader, speaker of the House, and majority and minority leaders. You should be aware, however, that below these higher levels of leadership, other party leaders exist, and they can wield significant power in terms of how bills move through Congress or a state legislature. Much of their power can be attributed to partisan politics—particularly the power that comes from the party holding the majority in each chamber (the House or the Senate).

Partisan is defined as "a firm adherent to a party, faction, cause, or person... political partisans who see only one side of the problem" (Partisan, n.d.). As citizens, we hope to elect officials to office who will serve as statesmen and women and who understand that their responsibility is to create laws to serve the common good. However, partisan agendas, campaign promises, and pressure from party leadership and powerful lobbying groups all have an impact on the policymaking process.

As discussed, the work of passing bills into laws happens at the committee level, so it is important to know how committees are structured, which legislators drive them, and how partisan politics works at this level—particularly with regard to moving the policymaking process along. Each committee is chaired by a legislator who represents the majority party. Each committee also has a vice chair—also from the majority party—who runs the business of the committee in the event the chair is unable. The senior member of the committee from the minority party serves as the minority party leader on that committee and is often known as the *ranking member*.

Understanding this—and noticing how partisan politics serves to enable or constrain the making of good policy—can empower advocacy groups in their efforts to leverage for change before the final steps of lawmaking have been achieved. Once a law is in effect, it is difficult to change.

> Understanding the structure and function of the legislative committee and the agenda of the majority party agenda, and preparing wisely before providing testimony or making any other type of appearance before a legislative committee, are both strategies to overcome challenges associated with the policymaking process.

The Importance of Cost

Although this is not a universal truth, policies often cost money to implement. If implementing a policy will cost the state or federal government money, that must be addressed, and future budget bills will need to appropriate funds. Examples of costs to consider in a fiscal analysis of a proposed policy include startup costs, training costs, and costs associated with changes in the structure of the regulatory agency affected by the policy. Cost estimates should also include either an ROI estimate or a cost-benefit analysis. An anticipated improvement in outcomes can be helpful in moving a policy that costs dollars along to fruition. Together, these considerations inform the decision by policymakers to adopt the proposed new policy or continue with the current practice.

If, however, legislation can be structured so it is cost-neutral, that can be an advantage for stakeholders attempting to advance the policy. An example of a cost-neutral policy is a recently passed state board of nursing program that provides for nursing education grants. This policy was planned so that it would be financially supported by a nominal increase in nursing licensure renewal fees (established in the law that created the grant program). Policymakers were also presented with data indicating how the grant program would affect affordability of further nursing education for nurses, nursing jobs, and growth in the healthcare industry. Evidence in the literature supporting progression in nursing education (from LPN to RN, from RN to BSN, and so on), plus cost-neutrality, made an impact on policymakers, and the measure passed the legislature.

Stakeholder Influence

A *stakeholder* is "one that has a stake in an enterprise" or "one who is involved in or affected by a course of action" (Stakeholder, n.d.). A stakeholder, therefore, may be any government actor, private citizen, or representative of an interest group with a stake in policymaking. Legislators, congressmen and women, executive branch and regulatory agency staff, special interest group lobbyists representing trade and professional organizations, advocacy group leaders, and individual citizens all constitute stakeholders. Their influence may depend on a number of factors, including their vote as a constituent, their power and influence on a statewide or national level, and most especially, their capacity to donate financially to political action committees and directly to political campaigns. Organizations with the most political capital are often those with the largest budgets focused on political leverage. However, lawmakers can also be moved by their constituents' individual stories if they are compelling.

Expert Opinion

Expert opinion on a matter of policy might be offered by a variety of actors, from individual scientists or teams who have conducted research on the matter, to clinicians or practitioners, to committees or commissions created and funded by US Congress or state legislatures to investigate a specific topic to inform a policy direction. It is common for experts in the field to provide testimony based on their own expertise; however, that testimony holds even greater leverage if they are authorized to represent an organization or state or federal commission. Expert opinion might also come in the form of guidelines and reports from reputable government or private organizations—for example, the CDC, the National Academy of Medicine (NAM), or a professional organization.

Expert opinion supported by rigorous research is often given serious consideration during the policymaking process, as it should be. This type of expert opinion might come into play in one of two ways:

- Written expert opinion level VII evidence—for example, reports from the CDC or NAM—may be used as part of the body of global evidence, which is discussed in Chapter 7, "The Foundation: Steps 0 Through 3."

- A more personal delivery of expert opinion by persons who are expert in their field—often with a body of evidence to support their dialogue or testimony—may occur. This type of expert opinion is even more powerful and provides greater leverage if the speaker has earned personal credibility over time and represents a credible organization.

Summary

This chapter discussed policymaking processes and models. When an idea for a new policy is formulated, it must go through specific procedures before it can be introduced as a bill and eventually become law. These procedures have been addressed in some detail. Additionally, once a bill has been enacted into law, it must be implemented, normally by a governmental agency. For this to happen, regulations are usually written to flesh out the legislative intent.

A variety of policy process frameworks and models exist that are helpful in understanding and advancing policymaking. Four of these were described: John Kingdon's streams model, Sabatier's Advocacy Coalition Framework, the CDC policy analytical framework, and force-field analysis, which developed from Lewin's field theory model. Finally, the chapter discussed how partisan politics, costs, stakeholders, and expert opinion influence the policymaking process.

References

Burnes, B., & Cook, B. (2013). Kurt Lewin's field theory: A review and re-evaluation. *International Journal of Management Reviews, 15*(4), 408–425.

Carey, M. P. (2013, June 17). *The federal rulemaking process: An overview.* Congressional Research Service Report R:32240. Retrieved from https://fas.org/sgp/crs/misc/RL32240.pdf

Center for Responsive Politics. (n.d.-a). American Medical Assn. Retrieved from https://www.opensecrets.org/orgs/summary.php?id=D000000068

Center for Responsive Politics. (n.d.-b). American Nurses Assn. Retrieved from https://www.opensecrets.org/lobby/clientsum.php?id=D000000173&year=2017

Center for Responsive Politics. (n.d.-c). Health sector profile, 2017. Retrieved from https://www.opensecrets.org/lobby/indus.php?id=H&year=2017

Centers for Disease Control and Prevention. (2013). CDC's policy analytical framework. Retrieved from https://www.cdc.gov/policy/analysis/process/analysis.html

Centers for Disease Control and Prevention, Office of the Associate Director for Policy. (2015). CDC policy process. Retrieved from https://www.cdc.gov/policy/analysis/process/index.html

Congress.gov. (n.d.-a). *The legislative process: Calendars and scheduling* [Video file]. Retrieved from https://www.congress.gov/legislative-process/calendars-and-scheduling

Congress.gov. (n.d.-b). *The legislative process: Committee consideration* [Video file]. Retrieved from https://www.congress.gov/legislative-process/committee-consideration

Congress.gov. (n.d.-c). *The legislative process: House floor* [Video file]. Retrieved from https://www.congress.gov/legislative-process/house-floor

Congress.gov. (n.d.-d). *The legislative process: Introduction and referral of bills* [Video file]. Retrieved from https://www.congress.gov/legislative-process/introduction-and-referral-of-bills

Congress.gov. (n.d.-e). *The legislative process: Presidential actions* [Video file]. Retrieved from https://www.congress.gov/legislative-process/presidential-action

Congress.gov. (n.d.-f). *The legislative process: Resolving differences* [Video file]. Retrieved from https://www.congress.gov/legislative-process/resolving-differences

Congress.gov. (n.d.-g). *The legislative process: Senate floor* [Video file]. Retrieved from https://www.congress.gov/legislative-process/senate-floor

Cordell, L. D. (2019). *Barriers to effective hyperglycemia management and clinical practice guideline adherence in the inpatient blood and marrow transplant population: An evidence-based guideline evaluation and intervention project* (Unpublished doctor of nursing practice project). The Ohio State University, Columbus, Ohio.

Disney Educational Productions. [YouTube]. (2011, Dec. 8). *Schoolhouse Rock: I'm Just a Bill* [Video file]. Retrieved from https://www.youtube.com/watch?v=FFroMQlKiag

Egan, T. (2004). *How a bill becomes a law*. New York, NY: Rosen Publishing Group.

GovTrack. (2018a). How a bill becomes a law. Retrieved from https://www.govtrack.us/how-a-bill-becomes-a-law

GovTrack. (2018b). Statistics and historical comparison. Retrieved from https://www.govtrack.us/congress/bills/statistics

Howlett, M., McConnell, A., & Perl, A. (2015). Streams and stages: Reconciling Kingdon and policy process theory. *European Journal of Political Research, 54*(3), 419–434. doi:10.1111/1475-6765.12064

Kingdon, J. W. (1995). *Agendas, alternatives, and public policies* (2nd ed.). Harlow, UK: Longman.

Lewin, K. (1939). Field theory and experiment in social psychology: Concepts and methods. *American Journal of Sociology, 44*(6), 868–896.

LexisNexis. (2007). House and Senate reports. Retrieved from https://www.lexisnexis.com/help/cu/TP/House_and_Senate_Reports.htm

Loversidge, J. M. (2019). Government response: Regulation. In J. A. Milstead & N. M. Short (Eds.), *Health policy & politics: A nurse's guide* (6th ed., pp. 57–86). Burlington, MA: Jones & Bartlett.

Magleby, D. B., Monroe, N. W., & Robinson, G. (2018). Amendment politics and agenda setting: A theory with evidence from the US House of Representatives. *Journal of Law, Economics, and Organization, 34*(1), 108–131. doi:10.1093/jleo/ewx016

Office of the Federal Register. (2011). *A guide to the rulemaking process*. Retrieved from https://www.federalregister.gov/uploads/2011/01/the_rulemaking_process.pdf

Office of the Legislative Counsel: US House of Representatives. (n.d.). HOLC guide to legislative drafting. Retrieved from https://legcounsel.house.gov/HOLC/Drafting_Legislation/Drafting_Guide.html

Office of the Legislative Counsel: US Senate. (n.d.). Responsibilities of the legislative drafter. Retrieved from https://www.slc.senate.gov/Drafting/drafting.htm

Partisan. (n.d.). In *Merriam-Webster's online dictionary*. Retrieved from https://www.merriam-webster.com/dictionary/partisan

Rambur, B. A. (2017). What's at stake in U.S. health reform: A guide to the Affordable Care Act and value-based care. *Policy, Politics & Nursing Practice, 18*(2), 61–71. doi:10.1177/1527154417720935

Rawat, P., & Morris, J. C. (2016). Kingdon's "streams" model at thirty: Still relevant in the 21st century? *Politics & Policy, 44*(4), 608–638. doi:10.1111/polp.12168

Regulations. (n.d.). In *The People's Law Dictionary*. Retrieved from https://dictionary.law.com/Default.aspx?selected=1771

Sabatier, P. A. (1988). An advocacy coalition framework of policy change and the role of policy-oriented learning therein. *Policy Sciences, 21*(2/3), 129–168.

Stakeholder. (n.d.). In *Merriam-Webster's online dictionary*. Retrieved from https://www.merriam-webster.com/dictionary/stakeholder

Swanson, D. J., & Creed, A. S. (2014). Sharpening the focus of force field analysis. *Journal of Change Management, 14*(1), 28–47. doi:10.1080/14697017.2013.788052

US Government Publishing Office. (n.d.). United States Statutes at Large. Retrieved from https://www.gpo.gov/fdsys/browse/collection.action?collectionCode=STATUTE

US House of Representatives Committee on Rules Majority Office. (n.d.). Discharge petitions. Retrieved from https://archives-democrats-rules.house.gov/archives/discharge_pet.htm

US House of Representatives: History, Art & Archives. (n.d.). Electronic voting machine. Retrieved from http://history.house.gov/Collection/Detail/42898

US Senate. (n.d.). Glossary term: Cloture. Retrieved from https://www.senate.gov/reference/glossary_term/cloture.htm

USA.gov. (2018). How laws are made and how to research them. Retrieved from https://www.usa.gov/how-laws-are-made

Weible, C. M., Sabatier, P. A., Jenkins-Smith, H. C., Nohrstedt, D., Henry, A. D., & deLeon, P. (2011). A quarter century of the advocacy coalition framework: An introduction to the special issue. *The Policy Studies Journal, 39*(3), 349–360. doi:10.1111/j.1541-0072.2011.00412.x

Weible, C. M., Sabatier, P. A., & McQueen, K. (2009). Themes and variations: Taking stock of the advocacy coalition framework. *The Policy Studies Journal, 37*(1), 121–140. doi:10.1111/j.1541-0072.2008.00299.x

"Absence of evidence is not evidence of absence."

–Carl Sagan

6

AN OVERVIEW OF AN EVIDENCE-INFORMED HEALTH POLICY MODEL FOR NURSING

–JACQUELINE M. LOVERSIDGE, PHD, RNC-AWHC

KEY CONTENT IN THIS CHAPTER

- Where does evidence fit in health policymaking?
- Comparing an evidence-informed health policy (EIHP) model and EBP models
- Components of EIHP and EBP models: a comparison
- The eight steps of an EIHP model

Where Does Evidence Fit in Health Policymaking?

That evidence-based practice (EBP) is the principal process used to address clinical problems is undisputed. The challenge for nurses and other healthcare providers involved in influencing and shaping policy and in supporting policymakers is to become skilled in applying the same kind of evidence-informed approach for maximum effect in that milieu.

Oxman, Lavis, Lewin, and Fretheim (2009) purport that an evidence-informed approach accomplishes several goals:

- It enables policymakers to be in command of their own use of the research evidence presented to them by expert stakeholders.

- It provides them with the ability to manage possible misuse of evidence by stakeholders, such as lobbyists or researchers, who are advocating for special-interest groups and therefore for specific policy positions.

- It enables them to approach policy development from a place of realism. A thorough understanding of the science underpinning a proposed policy allows the policymaker to appreciate that policy may be informed by less-than-perfect or incomplete information. For policymakers, this reduces political risk if a resulting policy is less than fully successful.

Understanding how policymakers might use evidence can be helpful when speculating about what kind of evidence to present and when and how to fit evidence into the policymaking process. The stronger the evidence that can be supplied to policymakers, the better the policy—at least in theory. In summary, an evidence-informed approach enables policymakers to (Oxman et al., 2009, p. 2):

- Ask critical questions about the research evidence available to support advocated policies.

- Demonstrate that they are using good information on which to base their decisions.

- Ensure that evaluations of their initiatives are appropriate and that the outcomes being measured are realistic and agreed upon in advance.

In addition to understanding the potentially supportive use of evidence in policymaking, it is imperative to appreciate how evidence fits into the process. With the increase of evidence-based policymaking in countries such as the UK, Australia, and the Netherlands, many scholars have conceptualized the use of evidence in policymaking as the ideal.

Cairney (2016) calls this point of view *comprehensive rationality*. He suggests applying a more realistic and useful approach called *bounded rationality*, which emphasizes the limits of the use of evidence and embraces the totality of the political environment in which policy is made (Cairney, 2016).

> In a best-case scenario, evidence provides lawmakers with the best research and other forms of information available to inform dialogue among stakeholders and provide leverage to achieve the best possible outcome.

Comparing an Evidence-Informed Health Policy (EIHP) Model and EBP Models

EBP models are process models. Regardless of which one is used, EBP models offer components and steps to guide the user in defining a clinical problem or issue and in identifying, critiquing, and synthesizing the evidence that will inform a logical response to that problem or issue. The EBP process also incorporates both clinical expertise and patient preferences and values. The end point of the EBP process is that a decision about how to address a clinical problem is reached. Quality-improvement projects, better clinical policies and procedures, and updated clinical guidelines are all results that rely on this process.

In evidence-informed policymaking, a similar process can be used. EBP models cannot be applied directly to policymaking, however, because of differences in purpose, stakeholders, and milieu. How a policy problem is defined, how the policy question is asked, and which categories of external or internal evidence will best inform policy options are all influenced by the policymaking environment. Additionally, there are no patients in the policy milieu; instead, there are citizens—the stakeholders typically most directly affected by the policy. So, although the process may be similar, the purpose, terms, uses of evidence, and contexts are different. As a result, to use EBP-like models in health policymaking, they must be adapted.

What follows in this and subsequent chapters is a guide to addressing health policy problems using an evidence-informed health policy (EIHP) model. This EIHP model was developed for use in nursing education and nursing regulation. However, its processes are general enough that it may be used to understand or advance health policymaking at the local, state, or federal level, by nurses or other health professionals, in environments beyond nursing education or nursing regulation. For example, the model has been successfully employed to retrospectively analyze existing regulatory policy—one of its intended uses (Damgaard & Young, 2017).

The EIHP model (Loversidge, 2016) is an adaptation of the Melnyk and Fineout-Overholt (2015) EBP model. Implementation of the Melnyk and Fineout-Overholt EBP model in organizations is described in the ARCC Model, but the EIHP adaptation is limited to modifications of the EBP model definition, the three major components, and the seven steps. Although other EBP models are adaptable to EIHP, the Melnyk and Fineout-Overholt EBP model (2015) was adapted for the purposes of this book for the following two reasons:

- Its three major components (external evidence, clinical expertise, and patient preferences and values) are compatible with like categories relevant to health policymaking.

- Its seven-step process is clear and focused and is adaptable to the policymaking process—as long as EIHP model users are cognizant of the policymaking process's nonlinear nature (Loversidge, 2016) and keep Cairney's (2016) principle of bounded rationality in mind. That is, the steps in the EIHP model might or might not occur in order, and when they do, they may spiral or circle back. (In evidence-informed policymaking, nonlinearity and complexity are process norms.)

Defining EBP and EIHP: A Review

Chapter 1, "Extending the Use of Evidence-Based Practice to Health Policymaking," defined EBP (Melnyk & Fineout-Overholt, 2015) and EIHP (Loversidge, 2016). For the purposes of review, these definitions are repeated here. Note the necessarily clinical focus of this EBP model and its three-pronged approach.

According to the Melnyk and Fineout-Overholt (2015) definition, EBP is:

- a paradigm and lifelong problem-solving approach to clinical decision making that involves the conscientious use of the best available evidence . . . with one's own clinical expertise and patient values and preferences to improve outcomes for individuals, groups, communities, and systems. (p. 604)

The definition of EIHP (Loversidge, 2016) is modified from that of EBP to allow for the necessary differences. Clinical expertise is replaced by expertise related to the policy problem or issue, and patient preferences and values are replaced by the values and ethics of the stakeholders who will be involved in the policymaking process. The intended outcome is also significantly different. By this definition, EIHP:

- combines the use of the best available evidence and issue expertise with stakeholder values and ethics to inform and leverage dialogue toward the best possible health policy agenda and improvements. (p. 27)

Components of EIHP and EBP Models: A Comparison

EBP models consist of three components (Melnyk & Fineout-Overholt, 2015, p. 4):

- **External evidence:** Sources of external evidence might include research, evidence-based theories, and evidence from opinion leaders or expert panels.

- **Clinical expertise:** This includes internal evidence generated from quality improvement or outcomes management projects, thorough assessment and evaluation of patients, and other available resources.

- **Patient preferences and values:** These include any concerns patients have regarding their clinical situation, treatment, and associated decisions and choices, and the values they hold.

The components of the EIHP model are parallel but adapted to the policy environment. They also exhibit language differences. The three major components of the EIHP model are as follows (Loversidge, 2016, p. 29):

- **External evidence:** External evidence in EIHP, as in EBP, consists of data that are generated from rigorous research. This includes research that is intended to be generalized to clinical settings and situations as well as policy research conducted on the national or global level and therefore considered global evidence. External evidence also includes evidence-informed relevant theories and best evidence from opinion leaders, expert panels, and relevant government and private data sources. Some of these evidence sources, including government and private data, might contribute what is known as *local evidence*. Chapter 7, "The Foundation: Steps 0 Through 3," provides a more complete explanation of global and local evidence sources.

- **Issue expertise:** This component focuses on expertise on the issue rather than the clinical problem. Issue expertise includes data from a variety of sources, such as professional associations, healthcare organizations, or government/executive branch agencies. Expertise also comes from experience professionals in the field might have with the policy issue. This may be gleaned from their testimony during legislative or regulation hearings or their work with professional associations in stakeholder meetings. Other issue expertise resources may be sought—for example, individuals who can provide expertise on matters related to quality and safety, practice, or consumer issues.

- **Stakeholder values and ethics:** This last component focuses on the values of stakeholders rather than of patients. Stakeholders might include healthcare providers, policy-shapers and policymakers, healthcare consumers, consumer-protection or interest groups, or healthcare organizations. Government agencies responsible for policy implementation may also be considered stakeholders.

Table 6.1 compares components of EBP and EIHP.

TABLE 6.1 A Comparison of EBP Components and EIHP Components

Evidence-Based Practice (EBP) Components	Evidence-Informed Health Policy (EIHP) Components
External evidence • Research • Evidence-based theories • Best evidence from opinion leaders and expert panels	**External evidence** • Best research evidence • Evidence-informed relevant theories • Best evidence from opinion leaders, expert panels, and relevant government and private data sources
Clinical expertise • Internal evidence generated from outcomes-management or quality-improvement project data • Patient-assessment or staff-survey data • Data from other types of organizational, departmental, or available resources	**Issue expertise** • Data from professional associations, healthcare organizations, or government agencies with policy implementation experience • Professions' understanding or experience with health policy issue—for example, data from professional associations or testimony • Other available resources or data related to potential quality and safety or practice or consumer issues
Patient values and preferences • Patients and partners in care	**Stakeholder values and ethics** • Healthcare providers • Policy shapers • Healthcare consumers and consumer-protection and interest groups • Healthcare organizations • Government agencies responsible for implementation • Other stakeholders

Components of the EIHP adapted from "The Components of EBP." Used with permission (Melnyk & Fineout-Overholt, 2015, p. 10).

Comparison of components of EBP and EIHP reprinted with permission from the Journal of Nursing Regulation *(Loversidge, 2016, p. 30).*

The components of EBP are conceptualized within the context of a supportive organizational culture and environment. The relevance of a supportive context is described in the Melnyk and Fineout-Overholt ARCC Model (2015). This supportive context enables the EBP process to actualize excellence in clinical decision-making and ultimately results in quality patient outcomes (Melnyk, 2017).

By comparison, the components of EIHP are conceptualized within the context of a political environment that includes a variety of interconnected systems and forces. These systems and forces are likely to be less supportive than those in organizations that support EBP. The policymaking environment may be supportive when lawmakers or other policymakers are working collaboratively with research scientists, professional association representatives, and others to ensure that policy is informed by the best research evidence and when the political agenda is aligned with research findings. At other times, the political environment may be less than supportive—even hostile—to the introduction of evidence that might intercede in the advancement of political agendas.

The success or failure of the application of good evidence to health policymaking depends on factors such as the values and political agendas inherent in partisan politics, the stance of powerful lobbies, legislative and budget cycles, and the always-present potential for the misinterpretation or misuse of evidence for political advantage. Lawmakers who sponsor a policy normally do what they can to pave the way for positive policy change, but the reality is that the environment is often less than supportive.

The Eight Steps of an EIHP Model

The seven steps of EBP begin with the cultivation of a spirit of inquiry. Then clinical questions are identified and addressed. The culmination of the EBP process is to integrate the three components of EBP—best evidence, clinical expertise, and patient preferences and values—to make a practice decision or change. The EBP decision or change outcomes are then evaluated and disseminated (Melnyk, 2017).

The eight steps of EIHP are comparable to the seven steps of EBP but are modified to focus on addressing health policy problems and serving within the context of a policymaking environment (Loversidge, 2016). The steps of the model are as follows:

0. Cultivate a spirit of inquiry in the policymaking culture or environment.

1. Ask the policy question in the PICOT format.

2. Search for and collect the most relevant best evidence.

3. Critically appraise the evidence.

4. Integrate the best evidence with issue expertise and stakeholder values and ethics.

5. Contribute to the health policy development and implementation process.

6. Frame the policy change for dissemination to the affected parties.

7. Evaluate the effectiveness of the policy change and disseminate findings.

Step 0: Cultivate a Spirit of Inquiry in the Policymaking Culture or Environment

This preliminary step of EIHP focuses on cultivating a spirit of inquiry within the policymaking culture or environment. During this step, attention is focused on the fact that a policy issue or problem needs to be addressed. Any number of actors might initiate or influence inquiry into the need for attention on a policy problem. These actors may include the following:

- **Individuals:** These include consumers of healthcare or individual healthcare professionals.

- **Special-interest groups:** In particular, this refers to health profession organizations or associations interested in seeking policy change. However, consumers with similar concerns may band together and form special-interest groups as well.

- **Lawmakers:** These actors might ask questions about the efficacy of certain healthcare programs, thus initiating inquiry out of the legislative branch of government.

Step 1: Ask the Policy Question in the PICOT Format

A key process step in EBP is to ask a relevant clinical question. This could be a background question or a foreground question. Background questions are broad, provide general information about a topic such as a condition test or treatment, and can be answered by looking to resources or textbooks. In contrast, foreground questions are very specific. When they are answered, they can provide evidence sufficient for making sound clinical decisions (University of Canberra Library, 2018).

When asking specific foreground clinical questions in EBP, the PICOT format is used. PICOT is an acronym for the elements of the question being asked. In EBP, PICOT stands for the following:

- Patient population of interest

- Intervention

- Comparison

- Outcome

- Time frame (optional)

> It is essential to structure a PICOT question appropriately to guide a search for evidence to inform the desired clinical practice change (Stillwell, Fineout-Overholt, Melnyk, & Williamson, 2010).

Asking and searching for answers to background and foreground questions are as important in health policymaking as in clinical decision-making. And, as with EBP, EIHP uses the PICOT approach. However, in EIHP, although PICOT still stands for patient population, intervention, comparison, outcome, and time frame, the meaning of most of these elements is different. This is because the question being asked is a policy question rather than a clinical one.

Note the differences in each of the EIHP PICOT elements (except for the time frame):

- **Population of interest:** In EIHP, the population of interest is composed of the consumers or constituents of a government policy—that is, citizens and residents or, more simply, people who will be affected by the policy change. There are some exceptions, however. For example, if a policy is focused solely on a category of professionals, those professionals might be the population of interest rather than citizens at large. This would be the case if, say, a proposed change will affect a licensure law—such as sections of a practice act that affect fees or disciplinary action—rather than the scope of practice (which would have an eventual effect on the care delivered to patients).

- **Intervention:** In the case of EIHP, intervention refers to the intended policy change—that is, what will be new or revised in law, regulation, or other policy.

- **Comparison:** With EIHP, comparison describes the status of the policy as it currently exists. Note that the comparison might indicate that policy is absent or lacking—that is, current policy is silent on the matter.

- **Outcome:** In the case of EIHP, outcome refers to the anticipated outcome after policy implementation.

- **Time frame:** As with EBP, in EIHP, specifying a time frame for achieving the outcome is optional.

> When the population (P), intervention (I), comparison (C), outcome (O), and time frame (T) are combined into a sentence, the policy issue or problem is synthesized and revealed (Loversidge, 2016).

Table 6.2 compares the PICOT elements as they are expressed in EBP and EIHP.

TABLE 6.2 A Comparison of EBP PICOT and EIHP PICOT

PICOT Element	EBP	EIHP
P	Patient/population of interest	Population of interest (citizen population, "persons-with," or a professional/licensed population)
I	Clinical intervention	Policy intervention (new or revised law, regulation, or other policy)
C	Clinical comparison	Comparison of what exists now in policy or whether policy is currently silent
O	Clinical outcome	Outcome following policy implementation
T	Time frame	Time frame

Using PICOT for Retrospective Analysis

As noted, in EBP, the purpose of asking a clinical question in PICOT is to enhance the efficiency with which the literature search will be accomplished. That is, the PICOT question guides and simplifies the literature search (Stillwell et al., 2010). The same is true in EIHP, except that it asks a policy question rather than a clinical question. However, in EIHP, the PICOT question may also serve a second purpose, which is to analyze an existing or pending policy by deconstructing it into its component parts (Loversidge, 2016). This is called *retrospective analysis.* Chapter 7 outlines the procedure for using the PICOT for retrospective analysis.

Step 2: Search For and Collect the Most Relevant Best Evidence

The next step in the process is a search in the literature for relevant evidence. In EBP, the purpose of asking a clinical question in PICOT is to enhance the efficiency with which this search will be accomplished. That is, you use keywords and synonyms from the PICOT question to conduct the search. This search necessitates the development of a search strategy to ensure appropriate research databases are explored.

Standard search strategies include:

- Querying multiple online research databases
- Using different combinations of keywords
- Identifying criteria and limitations of the search (for example, search only for resources published in the English language, limit the range of publication years, and search for peer-reviewed journals only)
- Recording the combinations of database explorations/keyword combinations
- Evaluating manuscript abstracts for appropriate content before downloading whole manuscripts for review

The goal of the literature search in EBP is to conduct a review comprehensive enough to obtain a body of evidence sufficient to inform a clinical practice change (Fineout-Overholt, Melnyk, Stillwell, & Williamson, 2010; Melnyk &

Fineout-Overholt, 2015). Similarly, the goal of the literature search in EIHP is to obtain a sufficient body of evidence to inform a policy change.

When searching for evidence, it is important to discern the difference between external evidence and internal evidence. In EBP, external evidence refers to research, evidence-based theories, and evidence from opinion leaders and expert panels (Melnyk & Fineout-Overholt, 2015). External evidence has a broader meaning in the policy environment, however. Therefore, in the EIHP model, external evidence also refers to evidence long held by policy researchers to be essential for informing policy—specifically, evidence from "relevant government and private data sources" (Loversidge, 2016, p. 29).

In EBP, internal evidence is "generated within a clinical practice setting from initiatives such as quality improvement, outcomes management, or EBP implementation projects" (Melnyk & Fineout-Overholt, 2015, p. 606); in the three-component model, internal evidence is categorized as clinical expertise. Internal evidence used in EIHP falls into the issue expertise component category. It might include data gleaned from professional associations, healthcare organizations, or government agencies; expertise provided by individuals familiar with the policy issue; or data and evidence obtained from other available and reliable sources not categorized as external evidence. More about the use of this type of evidence is described in the section on step 4; it is mentioned here to differentiate internal from external evidence.

Policy researchers refer to data that is relevant to policy but that does not otherwise constitute "research" on the evidence hierarchy as *local evidence* (Lewin et al., 2009):

> Local evidence is evidence that is available from the specific setting(s) in which a decision or action on an option will be taken. The word "local" in this instance can refer to district, regional or national levels, depending on the nature of the policy issue being considered. Such evidence might include information on the presence of factors that modify the impacts of a policy . . . [and] might include: the characteristics of an area and those who live or work in it; the need for services (prevalence, baseline risk or status); views and experiences; costs; political traditions; institutional capacity; and the availability of resources such as staff, equipment and drugs. (p. 2)

Data from external evidence of any type must be sound, reliable, and relevant if it is to be used to inform the policymaking dialogue (Loversidge, 2016).

Lawmakers may find that differentiating between external and internal evidence, while of importance to research scientists, is less important in policymaking, so long as the data are relevant to the issue and useful for informing the policy decision. Additionally, the search for evidence should seek to reveal any information that might clarify the problem. Concurrent developments relating to the extant policy problem, or political events, may be of great importance in directing, or redirecting, the search process.

Step 3: Critically Appraise the Evidence

It is important to use only research that will best inform the policy problem and to omit distracting and irrelevant information from the body of evidence (Loversidge, 2016). Therefore, after studies have been found that match keywords and synonyms, the full collection of articles should be summarized to identify those that are most likely to inform the policy problem. These are called *keeper studies.*

Keeper studies are systematically evaluated and synthesized using a process known as *critical appraisal,* which enables the evaluator to see similarities and differences between studies across the whole of the body of collected evidence. Using a spreadsheet or table is helpful in this process so that a record can be kept for each article. Recording the author and date of publication, the research design and methods, sampling, major variables, measurements used, data analysis techniques, researchers' findings, and any other notations will allow comparisons to be drawn (Fineout-Overholt et al., 2010). The level of evidence of each article is identified during this step, using the standard evidence hierarchy rating system (Melnyk & Fineout-Overholt, 2015). (For more on this system, refer to Chapter 2, "Using Evidence: The Changing Landscape in Health Policymaking.")

Step 4: Integrate the Best Evidence With Issue Expertise and Stakeholder Values and Ethics

In this step, the best evidence is integrated with the other two EIHP components: issue expertise and stakeholder values and ethics. The issue expertise component incorporates internal data—that is, data from sources such as professional associations, healthcare organizations, and key government agencies. This component also brings in expertise from individual health professionals. Issue expertise "acknowledges the professional wisdom of nurses and other point-of-care health professionals and their representative associations" (Loversidge, 2016, p. 29), making this step an ideal point at which nurses, generally representing their professional associations, should ensure their presence at the negotiating table if they have not been there from the start.

At this point in the process, engaging with other stakeholders may add momentum to the policy agenda (Loversidge, 2016). However, primary stakeholders should steel themselves for resistance and anticipate that the broad spectrum of stakeholder values and ethics will necessitate both dialogue and compromise at the negotiating table.

It is likely that this process will begin during the integration phase, and it will continue into step 5, during which the policy-development process is undertaken in earnest. Finally, other available resources might be sought for, or experts might come forward with, information or data related to quality and safety or consumer issues concerning the policy problem.

Step 5: Contribute to the Health Policy Development and Implementation Process

During this step, nurses and other healthcare providers contribute to the development and implementation of a viable policy option (Loversidge, 2016). Nurses and other healthcare providers are limited in their policymaking role. That is, their role is to advocate for a policy change and to provide evidence to advance the dialogue with lawmakers, regulatory agency staff, and other stakeholders. It is the lawmakers who have the power to sponsor bills and move them through the legislative process to make law. The rulemaking process is similar; executive branch regulatory agencies have legislative authority to write rules. Therefore, individual nurses, health professionals, and professional associations wishing to influence the process should engage with a variety of stakeholders, including lawmakers or regulatory agency officials, to contribute their expertise and command of the available body of evidence to the policy-development process.

Before a law or rule goes into effect is also a time to think about the implementation process, so that when the policy is enacted, implementation is realistic and meets the needs of constituents affected by the policy. Nurses and other healthcare providers can contribute to this planning process. Similarly, after a law is passed, the regulations needed to flesh out the details of the law will benefit from the implementation expertise provided by point-of-care practitioners.

Step 6: Frame the Policy Change for Dissemination to the Affected Parties

Step 6 of the EIHP model (Loversidge, 2016) represents a somewhat significant departure from Melnyk and Fineholt-Overholt's (2015) parallel step, which is to disseminate the outcomes of the EBP change. First, the results of policymaking in government contexts must be shared with the public they affect, and also must be implemented, before there are outcomes to be disseminated. Additionally, government policy is written in legal language. Therefore, in EIHP, before an enacted or finalized policy can be rolled out to the persons or groups it will affect, it should be framed, or summarized, so that constituents who will be affected by the policy will be able to understand the context and details of that policy. Dissemination should occur when policy is enacted but before it has gone into effect, so constituents are prepared when the policy takes effect. It is wise and appropriate to disseminate both a summary and the original language as enacted.

Step 7: Evaluate the Effectiveness of the Policy Change and Disseminate Findings

During this step, the success of the policy change and its implementation effectiveness is evaluated (Loversidge, 2016). Findings of that evaluation should be disseminated to parties affected by the change and to the public at large. Once a policy is in place, it is incumbent upon the government agency responsible for implementation to evaluate the effectiveness of the policy. However, this takes money, time, and human resources. Many agencies are underfunded, and if there is no allocation of resources to undertake the evaluation, then external evaluation is both possible and recommended. Often, agency data classified as public domain are sufficient in quantity for evaluation by an external private organization.

Table 6.3 compares the steps in EBP and EIHP.

TABLE 6.3   A Comparison of Steps in EBP and EIHP

Step	Steps of the EBP Process	Steps of the EIHP Process
0	Cultivate a spirit of inquiry within an EBP culture and environment.	Cultivate a spirit of inquiry in the policy culture and environment.
1	Ask the burning clinical question in PICOT format.	Identify the policy problem and ask the policy question in PICOT format.
2	Search for and collect the most relevant best evidence.	Search for and collect the most relevant best evidence.
3	Critically appraise the evidence.	Critically appraise the evidence.
4	Integrate the best evidence with one's clinical expertise and patient preferences and values in making a practice decision or change.	Integrate the best evidence with issue expertise and stakeholder values and ethics to make a health policy decision or change.
5	Evaluate the outcomes of the practice decision or change based on evidence.	Contribute to the health policy development and implementation process.
6	Disseminate the outcomes of the EBP decision or change.	Frame the policy change for appropriate dissemination to affected parties.
7		Evaluate the effectiveness of the policy change and disseminate the findings.

Steps of the EIHP process adapted from "The Steps of EBP." Used with permission (Melnyk & Fineout-Overholt, 2015, p. 10).

Comparison of steps of EBP and EIHP reprinted with permission from the Journal of Nursing Regulation (Loversidge, 2016, p. 30).

Summary

This chapter discussed where evidence fits in the health policymaking process. Nurses and other healthcare professionals on a quest to improve policy have the skills and resources to ask pointed health policy questions and contribute the best possible evidence and issue expertise to negotiate the best possible policy for themselves and their patients. Knowing how to search for and use evidence to move dialogue with lawmakers and other stakeholders increases the odds that policy will be based on evidence. Remembering that evidence-informed policymaking is an ideal, and that the totality of the political environment in which policy is made must be considered, will allow for a smoother journey through the process.

A useful map for nurses and other healthcare professionals to use on the evidence-informed policymaking journey is the evidence-informed health policy (EIHP) model. This chapter describes an EIHP model, adapted from the Melnyk and Fineout-Overholt EBP model (2015). Its components and steps were outlined and compared to EBP. Additionally, differences in the PICOT question to drive the literature search, and a second use for the PICOT question as a tool for retrospective analysis, were explained. The next three chapters describe each of the steps of the EIHP model in more detail.

References

Cairney, P. (2016). *The politics of evidence-based policy making*. London, UK: Palgrave Pivot.

Damgaard, G., & Young, L. (2017). Application of an evidence-informed health policy model for the decision to delegate insulin administration. *Journal of Nursing Regulation, 7*(4), 33–40. doi:10.1016/S2155-8256(17)30019-4

Fineout-Overholt, E., Melnyk, B. M., Stillwell, S. B., & Williamson, K. M. (2010). Evidence-based practice step by step: Critical appraisal of the evidence: Part I. *American Journal of Nursing, 110*(7), 47–52. doi:10.1097/01.NAJ.0000383935.22721.9

Lewin, S., Oxman, A. D., Lavis, J. N., Fretheim, A., Marti, S. G., & Munabi-Babigumira, S. (2009). SUPPORT tools for evidence-informed policymaking in health 11: Finding and using evidence about local conditions. *Health Research Policy and Systems, 7*(Suppl. 1), S11. doi:1186/1478-4505-7-S1-S11

Loversidge, J. M. (2016). An evidence-informed health policy model: Adapting evidence-based practice for nursing education and regulation. *Journal of Nursing Regulation, 7*(2), 27–33. doi:10.1016/S2155-8256(16)31075-4

Melnyk, B. M. (2017). The foundation for improving healthcare quality, patient outcomes, & costs with evidence-based practice. In B. M. Melnyk, L. Gallagher-Ford, & E. Fineout-Overholt (Eds.), *Implementing the evidence-based practice (EBP) competencies in healthcare: A practical guide for improving quality, safety, and outcomes.* Indianapolis, IN: Sigma Theta Tau International.

Melnyk, B. M., & Fineout-Overholt, E. (2015). *Evidence-based practice in nursing & healthcare: A guide to best practice* (3rd ed.). Philadelphia, PA: Lippincott Williams & Wilkins.

Oxman, A. D., Lavis, J. N., Lewin, S., & Fretheim, A. (2009). SUPPORT tools for evidence-informed health policymaking (STP) 1: What is evidence-informed policymaking? *Health Research Policy and Systems, 7*(Suppl. 1), S1. doi:10.1186/1478-4505-7-S1-S1

Stillwell, S. B., Fineout-Overholt, E., Melnyk, B. M., & Williamson, K. M. (2010). Evidence-based practice step by step: Asking the clinical question: A key step in evidence-based practice. *American Journal of Nursing, 110*(3), 58–61. doi:10.1097/01. NAJ.0000368959.11129.79

University of Canberra Library. (2018). Evidence-based practice in health. Retrieved from https://canberra.libguides.com/c.php?g=599346&p=4149723

"If I had an hour to solve a problem, I'd spend 55 minutes thinking about the problem and five minutes thinking about solutions."

–Albert Einstein

7

THE FOUNDATION: STEPS 0 THROUGH 3

–JACQUELINE M. LOVERSIDGE, PHD, RNC-AWHC

KEY CONTENT IN THIS CHAPTER

- Introduction to steps 0 through 3
- Step 0: Cultivate a spirit of inquiry in the policymaking culture or environment
- Step 1: Ask the policy question in the PICOT format
- Step 2: Search for and collect the most relevant best evidence
- Step 3: Critically appraise the evidence

Introduction to Steps 0 Through 3

As its title suggests, Chapter 6, "An Overview of an Evidence-Informed Health Policy Model for Nursing," provided an introduction and overview of an evidence-informed health policy (EIHP) model for nursing (Loversidge, 2016). This chapter provides more detail about the first four steps of the EIHP model:

- **Step 0:** Cultivate a spirit of inquiry in the policymaking culture or environment.
- **Step 1:** Ask the policy question in the PICOT format.
- **Step 2:** Search for and collect the most relevant best evidence.
- **Step 3:** Critically appraise the evidence.

Step 0: Cultivate a Spirit of Inquiry in the Policymaking Culture or Environment

Albert Einstein once said, "If I had an hour to solve a problem, I'd spend 55 minutes thinking about the problem and five minutes thinking about solutions." This is as true in policy as it is in theoretical physics. Thinking about a policy problem—considering it from all angles—is an essential requirement of the process at its early stages. Without this level of deep reflection, policy solutions may never come to light.

For this reason, step 0 of the EIHP model focuses on cultivating a spirit of inquiry in the policymaking environment or culture. This might occur during the legislative committee of a professional organization, a meeting of regulatory agency staff, or a conversation between legislators and their constituents.

> Of course, to be viable in the long run, policy options must have a likelihood of being realized during the implementation stage, meet the needs of key stakeholders, and align with partisan politics and political agendas. But to begin the process, it is sufficient to ask questions about policy problems and engage in dialogue in the spirit of inquiry.

Raising Inquiry

Is there a health problem that could be ameliorated by the institution of a suitable health policy? Could a "good" health policy improve a health problem indigenous to a certain population or region? If there is already a health policy, is there a problem with it as it currently exists? Maybe it is missing an essential component. Or perhaps it's too rigid or too flexible, making it less effective than it could be or difficult to enforce. These kinds of questions serve as springboards to discussion in a policy milieu and can stimulate people with common interests, missions, or goals to produce often ingenious options for addressing policy problems.

As discussed in Chapter 6, a variety of actors might stimulate this spirit of inquiry and ask good questions. These actors could include the following:

- **Individuals:** These include consumers of healthcare or individual healthcare professionals.

    - **Healthcare consumers:** This category of actors might call on their elected officials as individual constituents to ask to change a troublesome policy or generate a new policy, or could seek other consumers with like interests (described in the category special-interest groups, on the next page). For example, in recent years, constituents have approached their legislators about barriers to medication treatment imposed by third-party payers using a reimbursement protocol known as *fail first* or *step therapy*. This protocol limits insurance coverage of patient medications based on financial reasons rather than treatment efficacy. Under this protocol, a patient must try a medication selected by the insurer before he or she can use a more expensive medication prescribed by his or her provider—even if the more expensive drug is known to be more effective—putting the patient's health at risk. In one state, legislators introduced a bill limiting this practice. Without the initial conversation between various actors—in this case, the healthcare consumers who are the patients at risk and their elected officials—a viable policy solution would never have been reached.

    - **Individual healthcare professionals:** This cohort can also stimulate a spirit of inquiry. Of course, as citizens and constituents, private individuals have every right to voice their opinions and concerns to their legislators and regulators. However, it is generally more productive to work toward policy change within the context of one's professional association for two reasons. First, there is power in numbers. The best thinking and the most effective leverage usually arises from a body with some political capital. Second, it is usually in the best interests of both the profession and the citizens served to speak with one voice. When policymakers receive mixed or confusing input, it dilutes the message, which may be counterproductive—even at this early stage in the policymaking process.

- **Special-interest groups:** Special-interest groups form when policy concerns bring members together. Health professions organizations and healthcare consumers are the two most common categories of special-interest groups in the health arena.

  - **Healthcare consumer groups:** These usually have a particular policy focus or healthcare problem in common. They otherwise function as described previously; however, as with healthcare professionals, there is power in numbers.

    > Organized professional groups usually either seek or resist policy change, depending on their position, when an issue affects the care of the populations they serve or their scope of practice.

  - **Health professions organizations or associations:** These groups often seek policy change. Or, they may engage with lawmakers who, in the spirit of inquiry, ask questions about the efficacy of certain healthcare programs. National health professions associations lobby for policy change at the federal level, frequently interacting with members of the US Congress and federal regulatory agencies. State-level health professions associations do much the same thing at the state level—assuming they are large enough to support legislative committees, staff, or lobbyists. (It is often challenging for smaller state associations to work effectively in the state legislature, as a constant presence is helpful.) Regardless of how sophisticated these organizations are or what level of resources they can bring to bear, they should foster a spirit of inquiry by asking good questions about policies that could benefit from change and identifying problems that could benefit from new policy.

- **Lawmakers:** As discussed in Chapter 6, these actors might ask questions about the efficacy of certain healthcare programs, thus initiating inquiry out of the legislative branch of government. Lawmakers may have their own health policy agenda and might wish to leave a health policy legacy in state or federal law relative to an issue of some political urgency. For example, numerous lawmakers at both the state and federal levels have sparked inquiry to help them legislatively address the opioid crisis.

Formulating Background and Foreground Questions

In an environment that fosters a spirit of inquiry, a fundamental need to ask questions arises. Scholars have identified two types of useful questions for clinical problems; these categories also apply for health policy problems:

- **Background question:** This type of question asks for general knowledge (Dahlgren Memorial Library, 2018). In the clinical world, a background question generally pertains to a disease process, illness, or treatment and is a question for which the answer is likely available in a textbook or other general source. In the policy world, a background question might inquire about specific laws, rules, or other policies that exist on a topic of interest or about a legislative or regulatory process or rules of order.

- **Foreground question:** In a clinical environment, this type of question asks for specific knowledge to inform a clinical decision (Dahlgren Memorial Library, 2018). The foreground question is the basis for clinical questions based on the PICOT format. In the policy environment, the foreground question is the basis for the policy question based on the PICOT format.

Step 1: Ask the Policy Question in the PICOT Format

In clinical settings, the evidence-based practice (EBP) process begins when clinicians ask a question that directly relates to clinical practice. These questions surface as a result of inquiry; that is, the clinician notices a troublesome pattern, which evolves into a question. To find an answer to the question, the literature is searched for guidance. But without a plan, the search for answers may be derailed. A poorly planned search might yield too much or too little information, or the wrong kind of information, to help solve the clinical problem.

Using the PICOT format, which is a structure for formulating a targeted clinical question, can help researchers avoid these pitfalls (Melnyk & Fineout-Overholt, 2015; Stillwell, Fineout-Overholt, Melnyk, & Williamson, 2010). In policymaking, the PICOT format has much the same purpose. The difference is that PICOT asks a policy question rather than a clinical one.

To review, PICOT is an acronym for the elements of a question:

- **Population:** This refers to the population of interest—the consumer, citizen, or person who will be affected by the policy.

- **Intervention:** This is the intended policy change. This could be a new or revised law, regulation, or other policy.

- **Comparison:** This is the status of the policy as it exists currently.

- **Outcome:** This is the anticipated outcome following policy implementation.

- **Time frame:** This is the time frame for achieving the outcome. (It is optional.)

Combining the P, I, C, O, and T into a sentence synthesizes and reveals the issue (Loversidge, 2016).

Uses of PICOT Questions in Health Policymaking

In EBP, the PICOT question is formulated to focus and drive the literature search (Melnyk & Fineout-Overholt, 2015; Stillwell et al., 2010). The same is true in health policymaking: The PICOT question drives the literature search by identifying keywords to be used as search terms (Loversidge, 2016). However, policymaking rarely begins with a clean slate. It is not uncommon for policymaking to involve changes in existing policy—usually law or regulation. Therefore, a thorough analysis of what currently exists in these areas is essential before policy options can be developed.

Formulating a PICOT question based on existing (or pending) policy can be very helpful in the analysis process because it facilitates scrutiny of the existing or pending law or regulation (Loversidge, 2016). This process of retrospective (for an existing policy) or concurrent (for a pending policy) deconstruction helps in identifying who the policy affects and what the policy intends to accomplish and forces a closer look at the populations affected, intricacies associated with the intervention, and likelihood of efficacy of the intended outcome. A retrospective or concurrent analysis also allows for consideration of ethical and economic questions.

Asking a Focused Health Policy PICOT Question

It is essential to develop the skill to search for evidence to inform or analyze health policy by asking a well-designed health policy PICOT question.

When designing clinical PICOT questions, it is generally important to keep the PICOT parts as simple as possible. This is not always possible, or even desirable, when constructing a policy-related PICOT question. The complexity of the policy environment must be accounted for. If the PICOT question becomes too complex, it may be advantageous to formulate more than one to address various aspects of the health policy issue.

A policy PICOT question must be directly relevant to the issue or problem the policy intends to address and phrased so that it will direct the search for relevant information. The PICOT question should also clearly be about a policy. Healthcare providers who are accustomed to writing clinical PICOT questions tend to get lost in the clinical components of a PICOT question and may fail to explore important policy aspects.

Table 7.1 summarizes strategies for constructing the five elements of a PICOT question.

TABLE 7.1   Constructing a Policy PICOT Question

PICOT Element	Strategy
P (population of interest)	**Ask:** What is the population of interest? Start with the population and amplify the following: • **Citizens (country, state, city, county):** This applies depending on scope of legislation and whether the PICOT addresses a governmental policy. • **Patients:** This applies if the PICOT question addresses a patient-focused or organizational policy. Be precise and descriptive but brief. Note: There may be more than one population of stakeholders; the focus here is the population of citizens most affected by the intervention.
I (intervention)	**Ask:** What is the primary policy intervention being considered? Be specific. Make clear this intervention is in policy and is not a clinical intervention. Add as much detail as needed to drive the literature search, even if multiple search term combinations will be required.
C (comparison)	**Ask:** What is the alternative against which this policy compares? **Ask:** Does a policy currently exist? That is, is the intervention meant to revise an ineffective policy? **Ask:** Is there no policy against which to compare the intervention? (In this case, current policy is said to be *silent*.) The comparison describes what exists and generally points to the policy problem.

O (outcome)	**Ask:** Will the intervention (that is, the new or revised policy) affect the desired outcome for the target population?
	Be specific but also realistic.
	Avoid overdramatizing the potential outcome.
	The outcome must:
	• Relate directly back to the population (P)
	• Result from the intervention
T (time frame)	**Ask:** Is there a relevant time period that applies to the outcome?
	Ask: Does the time frame link back to the intervention?

Health Policy PICOT Question Template

To expedite research, templates for asking different types of clinical questions have been developed. Examples of such templates include PICOT question templates created by Fineout-Overholt (cited in Stillwell et al., 2010). Fineout-Overholt's templates differentiate between five types of clinical questions. The five types and their definitions are (Melnyk & Fineout-Overholt, 2015):

- **Intervention/therapy:** These ask what intervention or therapy will be most effective.

- **Prognosis/prediction:** These ask about indicators that are most predictive of or may carry the greatest risk for an outcome.

- **Diagnosis or diagnostic test:** These ask which assessments or tests will most accurately diagnose an outcome.

- **Etiology:** These ask about factors, processes, or conditions that are highly associated with outcomes (usually poor outcomes) and to what degree.

- **Meaning questions:** These ask how an experience might influence an outcome.

In the case of policymaking, a question about policy change—whether to institute a new policy or revise an existing one—constitutes an intervention.

Therefore, an intervention-type question template works best for constructing policy PICOT questions. I suggest the following template, which is a modification of the clinical EBP intervention template (Fineout-Overholt & Stillwell, 2015):

> For _____
> (P), how does _____
> (I), compared with
> _____ (C),
> affect _____ (O), in
> _____ (T)?

The word *affect* is used here because it is nondirectional; therefore, it will not bias a literature search. In contrast, words such as *improve, increase,* and *decrease* are directional. Using these types of directional words as key search terms limits your chances of reviewing literature that disconfirms a policy option that might otherwise appear to be a wise choice.

Strategy Tool 7.1: Sample PICOT Question: Telemedicine Health Benefits Bill

The delivery of healthcare using technology for remote examination, consultation, patient monitoring, and patient education is a boon to care, particularly in rural areas. However, as advances in telehealth services have been made across the country, an issue relating to healthcare reimbursement has come to the forefront.

In most states, telehealth services are covered by Medicaid. However, private health insurance payers are not necessarily required to cover telehealth, in spite of its established efficacy. In states that have not established requirements for private payers, this becomes a policy problem in that persons who are best cared for through telehealth services may need to pay out of pocket, go without healthcare, or travel long distances to access healthcare. Long-distance travel for some of these individuals could incur a financial burden, physical burden, or both.

To ameliorate this problem, a bill was introduced into a state legislature. Its PICOT elements were as follows:

Population: Persons receiving care via telehealth/telemedicine services.

Intervention: State law requiring health benefit plans/third-party payers to provide coverage for telehealth/telemedicine services on the same basis and to the same extent as in-person services.

Comparison: Current law is silent, which permits benefit plans to differentiate or omit coverage for telehealth/telemedicine services.

Outcome: Healthcare delivery efficacy, cost, and outcomes for the target population.

Note that no time frame is indicated. In a sentence, the PICOT reads as follows:

- For persons receiving care via telehealth/telemedicine services, how does state law requiring health benefit plans/third-party payers to provide coverage for telemedicine services on the same basis and to the same extent as in-person services, compared to current law, which is silent and permits benefit plans/third-party payers to differentiate or omit coverage for telehealth/telemedicine services, affect healthcare delivery efficacy, cost, and outcomes for the target population?

(Note that the terms *health benefit plans/third-party payers* are used in combination. This is because the bill used the term *health benefit plans,* but a quick search of the literature revealed that *third-party payers* is the more common term and therefore would be more useful in a search.)

After writing a PICOT question, you must ask whether it passes various tests:

- Is the population who will be most affected by this legislation readily identifiable?

- Is the intervention clear?

- Does the intervention relate directly to the population of interest?

- Is it clear that the intervention is a policy intervention, not a clinical intervention?

- Does the comparison describe what exists in policy at the present time—that is, before the bill was introduced?

- Does that comparison point to the policy problem?

- Is the outcome reasonable and clear, and does it relate to both the P and the I?

- Does the outcome avoid over-dramatization?

You must also ask whether the PICOT question includes words that can be used as key terms to drive the literature search. In this example, there are several terms that can be used:

- Telehealth or telemedicine (a quick search revealed these terms are index terms)

- Efficacy (or, as an alternative, efficiency)

- Cost

- Third-party payers

Strategy Tool 7.2: Differentiating Clinical and Health Policy PICOT Questions

As mentioned, the policy PICOT question should be written in such a way that it clearly addresses a policy problem rather than a clinical one. The following two examples demonstrate this distinction.

Example 1: Expedited Partner Therapy

Overview

Expedited partner therapy (EPT) is an accepted clinical practice. It involves treating sex partners of patients who have been diagnosed with certain sexually transmitted diseases (STDs), without examination, in an effort to prevent re-infection and minimize additional transmission (Centers for Disease Control and Prevention, [CDC], 2018).

Described as a Clinical Problem

Patients who present with and are treated for certain STDs are likely to be at risk for re-infection if their sex partners are not also treated. However, these sex partners may be unwilling or unable to seek treatment for their own infection.

Described as a Health Policy Problem

Patients who present with and are treated for certain STDs are likely to be at risk for re-infection if their sex partners are not also treated. The STDs in question are generally easily treated, and EPT is an accepted evidence-based treatment for which there are national guidelines. However, in some states, EPT is prohibited by law.

Written as a Health Policy PICOT Question

For persons diagnosed with certain STIs (STDs) and their sexual partners (P), how will state law permitting licensed prescribers to provide EPT by issuing a prescription or personally furnishing a drug for up to two sexual partners without examination (I), compared to pre-legislation practice, which prohibited EPT (C), affect incidence of infection/re-infection of the certain STIs and associated comorbidities (O) over a fiscal year state health department tracking period (T)?

Put the PICOT Question to the Test

- Is the population clear?

- Is the intervention detailed, and is it clear that it occurs in policy rather than in the clinical setting?

- Does the comparison point to the existing policy problem?

- Does the outcome relate directly back to the target populations? In this case there are two:

  - The person diagnosed with the STI

  - Up to two of that person's sexual partners

- Does the outcome result from the effect of the intervention, and is it realistic?

- Does the time period apply to the outcome and link back to the intervention?

Example 2: Meningococcal Disease Immunization

Overview

Meningococcal meningitis is a disease risk for young people. After babies and children under the age of 5, teenagers and first-year university students are especially at risk (Meningitis Now, n.d.). The CDC recommends that all 11- and 12-year-olds be vaccinated with meningo-coccal conjugate vaccine with a booster at age 16, and also that teens and young adults be vaccinated with a serogroup B meningococcal vaccine (CDC, 2017).

Described as a Clinical Problem

Young people, particularly those entering school systems, may come in contact with and be at a greater risk for contracting meningococcal meningitis. The CDC has identified recommended ages for vaccination and boosters. Parents and guardians of school-age children/minors, and primary-care/pediatric healthcare providers, should ensure that these young individuals are immunized against this preventable but potentially lethal disease.

Described as a Health Policy Problem

Young people, particularly those entering school systems, may come in contact with and be at a greater risk for contracting meningococcal meningitis. The CDC has identified recommended ages for vaccination and boosters. Immunization for virtually all communicable diseases is required for school-age children in accordance with CDC recommenda-tions. However, many states have not yet enacted policy in alignment with the more recent meningococcal meningitis immunization recom-mendations. State laws should require immunization for school-age children in accordance with these national guidelines.

Written as a Health Policy PICOT Question

For school-age pupils (P), how will state law requiring mandatory im-munization against meningococcal disease (I), compared with pre-legislation practice, which is silent on meningococcal immunization (C), affect the incidence of meningococcal disease in the target population (O) over a fiscal year state health department tracking period (T)?

Put the PICOT Question to the Test

You put this PICOT question to the same test as the previous one to facilitate the search for evidence. The logical process that is consistent across the two PICOT examples is that they both:

- Differentiate the health policy problem from the clinical prob-lem.

- Write the policy problem as a PICOT question.

- Put the PICOT question to the test.

Using the PICOT Question Retrospectively for Deconstruction and Analysis

As discussed, a PICOT question can be formulated about an existing or pending policy to facilitate the analysis process (Loversidge, 2016). This process of retrospective deconstruction involves partitioning the policy into its PICOT component parts by looking backward into the policy as it has been written rather than projecting how a literature search might inform the policy problem.

Strategy Tool 7.3: Example of a Retrospective PICOT Question

The extent and severity of the opioid crisis in the United States has stimulated lawmakers to attempt a variety of strategies to address this public health dilemma. It is known that the nonmedical use of prescription opioids may serve as a gateway to heroin use and that over-prescribing of opioids is a contributing factor (Compton, Jones, & Baldwin, 2016). One Midwest state's governor asked the regulatory agencies with oversight for prescribing healthcare professionals to jointly address opioid prescribing for acute pain. The boards of nursing, pharmacy, dentistry, and medicine agreed and promulgated rules that were consistent across the four boards. The focus of this analysis will be solely on the board of nursing prescribing regulations. A PICOT question focused on retrospective analysis of this regulation is as follows:

Population: Persons with acute pain.

Intervention: Prescribing of opioid analgesics limited to the following (The Ohio Board of Nursing, 2017):

- No more than seven days for adults.

- No more than five days for minors and only following written consent of parent/guardian.

- Providers may prescribe in excess of the day limit only if a specific reason is provided in the medical record.

- The total morphine equivalent dose (MED) cannot exceed an average of 30 MED per day.

- The limits do not apply to cancer, palliative care, end-of-life/hospice care, or MAT for addiction.

Comparison: No day or MED regulatory limits on opioid prescribing.

Outcome: Approximately 109 million fewer doses of prescribed opiates in Ohio (across the four boards of prescribers) that were not likely to have been needed by the person with acute pain for whom the limited dose was prescribed.

Time frame: Annual reduction in available opioid doses by nonmedical users; it was estimated that the rules, in effect since August 31, 2017, will reduce the number of doses that fall into the hands of nonmedical users in that state annually by 109 doses (Clark, 2017).

This PICOT articulates what the regulation does and who it affects. It is common to think about practice acts and regulations in terms of their effects on the practitioner or licensee, and it is true that these policies do have those effects. This rule requires prescribers to change their prescribing practices. However, it is the citizens with acute pain who are most affected by the prescribing limitations.

The state has a responsibility to protect the public. This translates to controlling the number of opioid doses available to people who need them and to people who might have access to a household in which prescription opioids are kept. The state must balance care of people with the desire to restrict opioid availability. The five-to-seven-day prescription range allows for coverage for a reasonable period of time—for example, a long or holiday weekend when the prescriber may not be reachable. For acute pain, this may also be a long enough period to test whether an additional course of treatment may be warranted without allowing for a surplus of the opioid prescription to be on hand in a household that might be accessible to a person at risk for opioid addiction. The rule also allows for exceptions; the prescriber may exceed the day limit if a specific reason is recorded in the medical record. In summary, partitioning this policy into its PICOT parts, retrospectively, allows for more thorough analysis.

The retrospective PICOT question should also meet the PICOT tests:

- The primary population of interest is the person with acute pain for whom the opioid is prescribed.

- The intervention is a regulation—a policy intervention rather than a clinical intervention—and focuses on how the prescribing relates back to the person with acute pain.

- The comparison describes what existed prior to the regulation, which was the absence of such a restriction.

- The outcome circles back to the person with acute pain, who will have a needed prescription but without surplus in the household.

- The time frame is a prediction, which was made public by state government officials in the news media, when the governor first discussed this initiative.

Step 2: Search For and Collect the Most Relevant Best Evidence

As discussed in Chapter 6, this step involves using keywords and synonyms from the PICOT question to conduct a thorough search for evidence. The goal is to conduct a comprehensive search so there is a sufficient body of evidence to inform health policy options and leverage dialogue. The range of external evidence to inform health policymaking includes research, evidence-based theories, and expert opinion, as well as relevant government and private data.

A thorough database search and comprehensive review of the literature is the normal procedure when searching for and collecting the most relevant best evidence (Melnyk & Fineout-Overholt, 2015). This is as important in EIHP as it is in EBP. However, differences in using evidence to inform health policymaking require a somewhat different approach. In policymaking, ensuring that the two types of evidence—global evidence and local evidence—are in balance is paramount.

Lewin, Oxman, Lavis, and Fretheim (2009) define *global evidence* as:

> the best evidence from around the world [and is] the best starting point for judgments about the effects of options and factors that modify those effects, and for developing insight into ways in which problems can be approached and addressed. (p. 2)

Alternatively, they define local evidence as:

> evidence that is available from the specific setting(s) in which a decision or action on an option will be taken [and] . . . can refer to district, regional or national levels, depending on the nature of the policy being considered. (p. 2)

Global Evidence: Systematic Reviews (and How and Where to Find Them)

Many argue that the most successful way to meet policymaker needs for global evidence is through the use of systematic reviews. The use of systematic reviews to help policymakers inform their decision-making has gained attention over the years, and efforts have been made to improve and support their use by health policymakers and decision-makers in health systems (Lavis, 2009; Lavis et al., 2005; Murthy et al., 2012).

By definition, systematic reviews seek to systematically, comprehensively, and exhaustively search for, appraise, and synthesize evidence obtained from research conducted by others. Typically, systematic reviews adhere to review conduct guidelines. They summarize what is known, offer recommendations based on what is known, and summarize what remains unknown. Additionally, any uncertainty around findings—as well as recommendations for future research—are reported (Duke University Medical Center Library & Archives [Duke], 2018).

Other types of reviews include literature reviews, meta-analysis, qualitative systematic review/qualitative evidence synthesis, systematized review, umbrella review, and others (Duke, 2018). Systematic reviews are the focus of this discussion, however. A key source of information in policymaking, systematic reviews offer the following advantages (Lavis et al., 2009):

- They reduce the likelihood of bias. Policymakers are less likely to be misled because systematic reviews are more transparent in the identification, selection, appraisal, and synthesis of research studies.

- They increase confidence in the precision of policy decision-making because they provide a larger number of units of study.

- They enable policymakers to focus on applying the findings of the systematic review to the policy problem rather than on the process of locating, appraising, and synthesizing evidence on their own.

- They allow stakeholders—including the public—to contest the evidence in a more constructive manner because it is presented in the systematic review in a more organized and transparent way.

A combination of keywords or phrases from the PICOT question may be used to conduct the search. Evidence from any level of the evidence pyramid may be used to inform health policymaking. However, keep in mind that retrieving a body of single studies will require individual appraisal and synthesis of the body of evidence, whereas a well-done systematic review focused on the policy problem will more likely have met those criteria.

Systematic reviews can be retrieved from any of the following databases:

- **The Cochrane Database of Systematic Reviews and the Database of Abstracts of Reviews of Effects:** Both of these are found in the Cochrane Library and accessed through the Cochrane Collaboration website, https://www.cochrane.org/.

- **McMaster Health Forum/Find Evidence:** A Canadian institution, the McMaster Health Forum is a World Health Organization (WHO) collaborating centre for evidence-informed policy. It offers a free online repository of pre-appraised and synthesized research evidence for health systems and for social-system policymaking at https://www.mcmasterforum.org/find-evidence/overview.

- **Hinari:** This program was established cooperatively by the WHO and various major publishers. It enables low- and middle-income countries to access one of the world's largest collections of health and biomedical literature. A list of eligible countries is found on the website's home page at http://www.who.int/hinari/en/.

- **PubMed:** This resource, available at https://www.ncbi.nlm.nih.gov/pubmed, includes MEDLINE, which contains journal citations and abstracts for literature of a biomedical nature from around the globe. (Visit https://www.ncbi.nlm.nih.gov/pubmed/clinical to see how to use the hedge filter to access systematic reviews.)

Strategy Tool 7.4: Using PICOT Keywords in a Systematic Review Search

The PICOT question from "Example 2: Meningococcal Disease Immunization" in Strategy Tool 7.2, "Differentiating Clinical and Health Policy PICOT Questions," was used to drive a search for systematic reviews using PubMed and the hedge filter instructions for accessing systematic reviews.

An advanced search using the terms *systematic review, meningococcal meningitis, vaccine,* and *prevention,* which were combined using the Boolean AND term, yielded 337 search results. Of these, only the first three were systematic reviews. However, all three appeared to be worth reading, as they were focused on the efficacy of the meningococcal vaccine and would be helpful in explaining the usefulness of the vaccine to policymakers. Other articles in the list of 337 search results were also scanned to determine whether they would inform a policy option in this matter. In addition, a second advanced search using the terms *systematic review, meningococcal vaccine,* and *state law,* combined using the Boolean AND term, revealed a single but relevant study critiquing criteria for evaluating vaccines for inclusion in mandatory school immunization programs.

The literature search should not exclude single studies. Although there are significant advantages to using systematic reviews to inform policy options, single studies have their use as well. For example, consider the PICOT question describing expedited partner therapy (EPT) in "Example 1: Expedited Partner Therapy" in Strategy Tool 7.2. A keyword search for systematic reviews is likely to discover national evidence-based EPT guidelines, but a different combination of keywords, including the word *policy* or *mandates,* reveals a different body of literature focused on state laws permitting EPT rather than on clinical guidelines. The word *mandate* is an indexing word that substitutes for the word *law* or *regulation.* Both search approaches are needed to inform the EPT policy dialogue.

Experimenting with PICOT keywords is important because research databases use an indexing language or controlled vocabulary. When a keyword is entered into a particular database, it is matched to its controlled vocabulary, and all articles with that topic can then be found using that one index term. A researcher will often need to determine which index term is closest to the keyword in terms of meaning. This is a time-saving technique and will ensure complete coverage (Stillwell et al., 2010).

Local Evidence: Where It Is and How It Is Appraised

Local evidence is useful at all stages of the policy process. It may position an issue on the policy agenda or be used by stakeholders and interest groups to advance a particular policy option. It can be particularly useful for estimating the magnitude of the problem, on a local level, that the policy aims to address. It can add detail that will be important to the economic impact or government delivery during policy rollout; inform the need for or availability of necessary human, technical, and infrastructure resources; and reveal potential barriers to policy implementation (Lewin et al., 2009).

Local evidence may be obtained from any number of sources, including the following:

- **Routine data:** This includes data about disease prevalence, cost of services, and utilization of healthcare.

- **Survey data:** This includes health statistics, demographics, and socio-economic conditions.

- **One-off studies:** These include locally conducted studies of consumer views on health issues.

The use of local evidence has advantages and disadvantages. While it may be more directly relevant to policymaking at a local or state level than studies that have been conducted elsewhere or with a less targeted aim in mind, it may also be less reliable. Even when the reliability of local evaluations is ensured, the results may be misleading (Lewin et al., 2009). Lewin and colleagues (2009) suggest that policymakers and those guiding them consider five questions to identify relevant and appropriate local evidence (pp. 4–11):

- **What local evidence is needed to inform a decision about options?** The evidence needed will depend on the policy option being considered, the context, and evidence availability.

- **How can the necessary local evidence be found?** The authors suggest that this type of evidence may be obtained from routine health information systems, from larger studies that can be disaggregated, or from specific studies that have been conducted on a local level. They caution against selectively using local evidence, or cherry-picking, because it may cause you to overlook important data.

- **How should the quality of the available local evidence be assessed?**
  Quality should be assessed to ensure that interpretation will be accurate. Several key questions can facilitate in this evaluation:

  - **Is the evidence representative?** That is, is the description of the evidence source clear, and is the evidence drawn from a sample composed of the population of interest? Also, is the description of how sampling was conducted clear, and was sampling conducted in an appropriate manner? Finally, does the evidence make inferences or generalizations regarding the wider population?

  - **Is the evidence accurate?** In other words, is data collection described and appropriate? Was data collection monitored? Was the method of analysis reported clearly? Were limitations discussed?

  - **Are appropriate outcomes reported?** That is, are the measures reported in the data a match for addressing the policy question for which the data will be used?

- **Are there important variations in the availability, quality, or results of local evidence?** In other words, are there variations in availability across geographic areas, jurisdictions, or population groups? If data are available from only one source and a cross-check is not possible, is there another way to determine reliability? Is the data available on a routine basis (for example, annually) or only one time, making for a noncomparable data pool?

- **How should local evidence be incorporated with other information?**
  Policy decisions are best informed by combining global evidence and local evidence. Together these comprise what is described as *external evidence*. The authors suggest that when local evidence might provide significant influence in decision-making, it is important to do the following:

  - **Describe the approach used to identify local evidence:** This is ideally a systematic approach.

  - **Describe the approach used to assess the local evidence:** If shortcuts or assumptions were necessary in the assessment, these should be made transparent.

- **Describe what local evidence is used and its sources:** Details about the specific groups or communities from which the evidence was obtained should be included and its sources cited.

- **Identify and describe important gaps or uncertainties because of a lack of local data or because of poor quality data:** It may be difficult to make decisions based on information if uncertainties are identified or data are of poor quality.

- **Identify and discuss differences between the findings obtained from the global evidence and the findings obtained from the local evidence:** Global evidence may be strong and compelling, but local evidence may suggest that a policy direction that has worked on a global scale may be less effective at the local level. The balance between local and global evidence must be appreciated, and whatever is likely to be most effective should be utilized.

> It is important to understand and communicate that local needs regarding evidence may be different from national or global needs—especially for issues such as health disparities, which are affected by geopolitical boundaries.

Step 3: Critically Appraise the Evidence

As described briefly in Chapter 6, after you collect evidence, you undergo rapid critical appraisal (RCA), a process of critically appraising that evidence, retaining only the research that best informs the policy problem (Loversidge, 2016). From the full collection of articles found using various keyword combinations, you review all *keeper studies*—that is, those studies most likely to inform the policy problem—to determine their level of evidence on the evidence hierarchy or pyramid (described in Chapter 1, "Extending the Use of Evidence-Based Practice to Health Policymaking").

As you appraise the evidence, you can use critical appraisal checklists. The checklist you use should be specific to the research methodology. Still, several general and preliminary questions may be asked. An excellent checklist gleaned from the use of critical appraisal for quantitative evidence in EBP follows (O'Mathuna & Fineout-Overholt, 2015). (Note that the last question is modified from a clinical practice problem to a policy problem.)

- **Why was the study done?** The researchers should clearly explain the study's purpose.

- **What is the sample size?** The sample should be described and should be sufficient to ensure confidence in the results and the effect demonstrated. Be aware that the methodology determines adequacy of sample size—that is, a much larger sample is required for a quantitative study, such as a randomized controlled trial, than for a qualitative study exploring the lived experience, as in phenomenological research.

- **Are the measurements of major variables valid and reliable?** In this section of a study, the concepts of validity and reliability should describe how an instrument measures a concept.

- **How were data analyzed?** Quantitative research reports should include the statistical tests used to analyze data. Qualitative research reports should clearly indicate what methods were used to analyze data.

- **Were there any untoward events during the conduct of the study?** If any problems occurred during the study, these should be reported, and if they affected the final results, this should be indicated.

- **How do the results fit with previous research in the area?** Study results generally fit into a growing body of evidence unless the researcher is exploring an area of study that is completely new. How the research expands on current knowledge—that is, what the study adds to the body of evidence—should be described.

- **What does this research mean for the policy problem?** The end goal of critical appraisal is to apply research findings to the policy problem. The question of how the study is relevant to the policy problem should be synthesized and established.

The language used for critical appraisal of qualitative evidence is somewhat different. An excellent checklist, also designed for use in EBP, is summarized here (Powers, 2015). (Note that the final question in this checklist is modified for use in policymaking.)

- **Are the results valid/trustworthy and credible?** This includes an assessment of how the study participants were chosen, how accuracy and completeness of data were ensured, and whether the description of the results is plausible and believable.

- **Are implications of the research stated?** Any new insights gleaned from the research should be assessed.

- **What were the study results?** Describe the results and how they fit the study's purpose.

- **Does the researcher identify the study approach?** As part of this assessment, indicate whether language, concepts, and methods—including data collection and analysis—are consistent with the approach.

- **Is the significance or importance of the study explicit?** Assess whether the literature review and/or description of the problem supports the need for the study.

- **Is the sampling strategy clear and consistent with study needs?** The researcher should clearly describe, justify, and control the sampling strategy, and the sample should reflect the study needs.

- **Are data collection procedures clear?** Assess whether the resource cites the data resources used and the means of verifying data, and explains researcher roles and activities.

- **Are data analysis procedures described?** Assess whether the analysis procedure(s) guides the sampling direction, whether data-management processes are described, and whether results are described and interpreted.

- **How are findings presented?** The presentation of findings should be logical and easy to follow. The presentation of data should use participant quotes when appropriate and should fit with the findings presented.

- **How are overall findings presented?** You should be able to derive meaning from the data, and findings should be presented in such a way that is understandable to readers.

- **How will the results inform the policy problem?** Determine whether the participant's experience and the presentation of findings could potentially have an impact on the policy dialogue.

Systematic reviews of the literature or meta-analyses may be particularly useful for leveraging a health policy dialogue, as discussed. In a systematic review, evidence on a particular topic has been systematically identified, appraised, and summarized according to criteria predetermined by the authors. Systematic reviews may incorporate meta-analysis but do not need to. A *meta-analysis* is a statistical technique used to summarize the results of a number of studies into one estimate; this gives more weight to larger studies (Oxman, Cook, & Gyuatt, 1994). Appraising these types of reviews requires a different procedure.

Oxman and colleagues' classic 1994 article provides guidance for appraising systematic reviews and/or meta-analyses. (Again, these steps have been summarized and slightly adapted for use in health policymaking.)

- **Did the overview address a focused question?** Unless the overview states an explicit question, you are left to guess whether it is pertinent to the policymaking question.

- **Were the criteria used to select articles for inclusion appropriate?** The authors must be clear on the criteria they used to select—and exclude—the research that was reviewed. Information about patients/subjects, exposures, outcomes of interest, methodological standards, and other details of interest should be scrutinized.

- **Is it unlikely that important relevant studies were missed?** The methods used by the authors to conduct the search should include a complete search of bibliographic databases, as well as a "hand search" of reference lists. In addition, personal contact with content experts is advised.

- **Was the validity of the included studies appraised?** Regardless of the types of studies included in the review, it is important to know if they were of good quality. The fact that the research was published in a peer-reviewed journal is in and of itself insufficient.

- **Were assessments of studies reproducible?** Review article authors make important decisions about which studies to include, how valid these studies are, and which data to extract from a particular study. These decisions require judgment. Generally, two or more people participate in these decisions, which guards against error. Agreement should be evident among the reviewers.

- **What are the overall results of the review, and how precise were the results?** The results of the review are often reported thematically; they should be clear and understandable. The reader should understand how precisely the effects can be applied to general populations (if applicable).

- **Will the results be relevant to the policy dialogue?** Questions to consider are whether the results can be applied directly to the policy problem and whether the benefits of applying the results of the systematic review are worth any potential harms or costs.

To determine the degree to which confidence should be placed in a systematic review to inform health policy, consider the following (Lewin et al., 2009):

- Did the review specifically address a policy or management question?

- Were criteria used for considering studies for the review that were appropriate and rigorous?

- Was the search for studies described in detail, and was it comprehensive?

- Were the studies assessed for relevance to the review topic—that is, did they meet inclusion criteria—and was each study's risk of bias transparent and reproducible?

- Were the results across studies similar?

The final step in RCA is to synthesize the evidence—that is, to look for similarities and differences across the whole of the body of available evidence. Once this is accomplished for the body of global evidence, the synthesis should be evaluated against a synthesis of comparable relevant local evidence.

This provided an overview of RCAs of quantitative and qualitative research and of systematic reviews. You might be able to adapt guidelines or checklists for EBP for use in EIHP. Sample RCA checklists for specific types of studies are available in the appendixes in *Evidence-Based Practice in Nursing and Healthcare: A Guide to Best Practice* (3rd edition), by Melnyk and Fineout-Overholt. Just keep in mind that your purpose is to appraise the evidence for its use in addressing a policy problem rather than a clinical problem.

Framing the Appraisal: Bridging the Gap Between Scientist and Policymaker

After you synthesize the body of global evidence and evaluate it against a synthesis of comparable relevant local evidence, you should prepare a summary report of both that will meet the needs of policymakers. To bridge the gap between scientists, researchers, or healthcare providers and other stakeholders, you must frame these findings so that policymakers both understand them and find them compelling. Here are some practical tips for framing and communicating a synthesis of evidence:

- **Build credibility:** You must build credibility with policymakers over time. If a research project is designed to inform a particular policy program, you will be better able to influence policymakers if communication between researchers and policymakers is continuous from the beginning of the project rather than waiting until the project is complete.

- **Package and present evidence:** Assemble the evidence to make systematic reviews less challenging for policymakers to understand. Evidence should be presented in a way that is accessible to policymakers but not oversimplified or distorted. Here are some ways to achieve this:

  - Provide a one-page summary of key messages (the synthesis).

  - Package and frame evidence in a way that ensures that all sections are covered. (For example, if you name three elements, cover all three elements.)

  - Be concise and clear in your presentation of findings.

  - Avoid jargon.

  - Be honest. Your message should be fully truthful and transparent. If policymakers or other stakeholders detect even a whiff of falsehood, all information will be discredited, as will you.

  - Use engaging visuals.

  - End with clear, specific, actionable recommendations that are context-specific and tailored to the needs of the target audience.

- Create a written three-to-four-page policy brief in the format that is most appealing to the target audience of policymakers and that will consume no more than 30 to 60 minutes of their time.

- Create a technical report, including a cover summary, if policymakers request a longer document with more complexity and detail.

- Create presentations and videos for consumption by policymakers.

Adapted from Pittore, Meeker, & Barker, 2017.

Summary

This chapter discussed the first three steps of the EIHP process. The first step, step 0, begins with the cultivation of a spirit of inquiry in the policymaking culture or environment. During this step, a policy problem or issue is identified.

In step 1, a question describing the policy problem or issue in the PICOT format is asked. After the question is asked, keywords from the PICOT question are used in step 2 to drive a search of the literature to collect the most relevant and best evidence. In policymaking, it is important to collect both global evidence (evidence from research studies) and local evidence. The PICOT question can also be used to retrospectively deconstruct an existing or pending policy for more thorough analysis.

In step 3, a process of rapid critical appraisal is undertaken to evaluate the evidence for its relevance and usefulness for informing a policy option. The most relevant best evidence is then synthesized. To be useful in policymaking, this synthesized evidence should be framed to bridge the gap between scientists, researchers, or healthcare providers and policymakers. It is essential that policymakers understand the results and implications of the evidence synthesis and its applicability to the policy option.

References

Centers for Disease Control and Prevention. (2017). Meningococcal vaccination. Retrieved from https://www.cdc.gov/vaccines/vpd/mening/index.html

Centers for Disease Control and Prevention. (2018). Expedited partner therapy. Retrieved from https://www.cdc.gov/std/ept/default.htm

Clark, J. (2017, Aug. 31). New limits take effect for opioid prescriptions in Ohio. *NBC4i. com.* Retrieved from https://www.nbc4i.com/news/new-limits-take-effect-for-opioid-prescriptions-in-ohio/1064641148

Compton, W. M., Jones, C. M., & Baldwin, G. T. (2016). Relationship between nonmedical prescription-opioid use and heroin use. *The New England Journal of Medicine, 374*(2), 154–163. doi:10.1056/NEJMra1508490

Dahlgren Memorial Library. (2018). Types of clinical questions. Retrieved from http://guides.dml.georgetown.edu/ebm/ebmclinicalquestions

Duke University Medical Center Library & Archives. (2018). Systematic reviews: The process: Types of reviews. Retrieved from https://guides.mclibrary.duke.edu/sysreview/types

Fineout-Overholt, E., & Stillwell, S. B. (2015). Asking compelling, clinical questions. In B. M. Melnyk & E. Fineout-Overholt (Eds.), *Evidence-based practice in nursing & healthcare: A guide to practice* (3rd ed., pp. 24–39). Philadelphia, PA: Lippincott Williams & Wilkins.

Lavis, J. N. (2009). How can we support the use of systematic reviews in policymaking? *PLoS Medicine, 6*(11), 1–6. doi:10.1371/journal.pmed.1000141

Lavis, J., Davies, H., Oxman, A., Denis, J. L., Golden-Biddle, K., & Ferlie, E. (2005). Towards systematic reviews that inform health care management and policy-making. *Journal of Health Services Research and Policy, 10*(Suppl. 1), 35–48.

Lavis, J. N., Oxman, A. D., Grimshaw, J., Johansen, M., Boyko, J. A., Lewin, S., & Fretheim, A. (2009). SUPPORT tools for evidence-informed health policymaking (STP) 7: Finding systematic reviews. *Health Research Policy and Systems, 7*(Suppl. 1), S7. doi:10.1186/1478-4505-7-S1-S7

Lewin, S., Oxman, A. D., Lavis, J. N., & Fretheim, A. (2009). SUPPORT tools for evidence-informed health policymaking (STP) 8: Deciding how much confidence to place in a systematic review. *Health Research Policy and Systems, 7*(Suppl. 1), 58. doi:10.1186/1478-4505-7-S1-S8

Loversidge, J. M. (2016). An evidence-informed health policy model: Adapting evidence-based practice for nursing education and regulation. *Journal of Nursing Regulation, 7*(2), 27–33. doi:10.1016/S2155-8256(16)31075-4

Melnyk, B. M., & Fineout-Overholt, E. (2015). *Evidence-based practice in nursing and healthcare: A guide to best practice* (3rd ed.). Philadelphia, PA: Lippincott Williams & Wilkins.

Meningitis Now. (n.d.). Meningitis in children and young people. Retrieved from https://www.meningitisnow.org/meningitis-explained/signs-and-symptoms/meningitis-children-and-young-people/#who-is-at-risk

Murthy, L., Shepperd, S., Clarke, M. J., Garner, S. E., Lavis, J. N., Perrier, L., . . . Straus, S. E. (2012). Interventions to improve the use of systematic reviews in decision-making by health systems managers, policy makers and clinicians. *Cochrane Database of Systematic Reviews, 12*(9). doi:10.1002/14651858.CD009401.pub2

The Ohio Board of Nursing. (2017). New limits on prescription opioids for acute pain. Retrieved from http://www.nursing.ohio.gov/PDFS/AdvPractice/New_Limits_on_Prescription_Opioids_for_Acute_Pain-Updated.pdf

O'Mathuna, D. P., & Fineout-Overholt, E. (2015). Critically appraising quantitative evidence for clinical decision making. In B. M. Melnyk & E. Fineout-Overholt (Eds.), *Evidence-based practice in nursing & healthcare: A guide to best practice* (3rd ed., pp. 87–138). Philadelphia, PA: Lippincott Williams & Wilkins.

Oxman, A. D., Cook, D. J., & Gyuatt, G. H. (1994). Users' guides to the medical literature: VI. How to use an overview. *Journal of the American Medical Association, 272*(17), 1367–1371. Retrieved from https://www.hopkinsmedicine.org/gim/_pdf/JAMA/6-Overview.pdf

Pittore, K., Meeker, J., & Barker, T. (2017). Practical considerations for communicating evidence to policymakers: Identifying best practices for conveying research findings. National Information Platforms for Nutrition. Retrieved from http://www.nipn-nutrition-platforms.org/IMG/pdf/communicating-evidence-to-policy-makers.pdf

Powers, B. A. (2015). Critically appraising qualitative evidence for clinical decision making. In B. M. Melnyk & E. Fineout-Overholt (Eds.), *Evidence-based practice in nursing & healthcare: A guide to best practice* (3rd ed., pp. 139–189). Philadelphia, PA: Lippincott Williams & Wilkins.

Stillwell, S. B., Fineout-Overholt, E., Melnyk, B. M., & Williamson, K. M. (2010). Evidence-based practice step by step: Asking the clinical question: A key step in evidence-based practice. *American Journal of Nursing, 110*(3), 58–67.

*"Design is not just what it looks like and feels like.
Design is how it works."*

–Steve Jobs

8

POLICY PRODUCTION: STEPS 4 AND 5

–JACQUELINE M. LOVERSIDGE, PHD, RNC-AWHC

Introduction to Steps 4 and 5

Chapter 6, "An Overview of an Evidence-Informed Health Policy Model for Nursing," briefly described steps 4 and 5 of the evidence-informed health policy (EIHP) model. The steps are as follows:

- **Step 4:** Integrate the best evidence with issue expertise and stakeholder values and ethics

- **Step 5:** Contribute to the health policy development and implementation process

This chapter discusses both steps more fully.

Of course, both steps are important to the EIHP process, but step 4—during which time the best evidence is integrated with issue expertise and stakeholder values—is particularly critical to the decision-making process. The goal of this step is to reach a decision about the next best steps in making a health policy change. One should think of this as a decision point in what is often a spiral, nonlinear process rather than an end point. Until a policy is enacted, there is always room for dialogue and always the possibility for change.

Integrating best evidence requires an understanding of two essential factors:

- The audience or stakeholders who will receive the evidence information summary

- The relevance of the evidence provided to that audience to policy at the local level

Recall from Chapter 7, "The Foundation: Steps 0 Through 3," that a combination of global and local evidence is used to inform dialogue and the policy decision. At the end of the day, however, policy must apply at the local level—which, in the United States, could be municipal, state, or federal—as defined by policymakers. (If outside the US, the local level will refer to the country or region within a country to which the policy will apply.)

Researchers and their representatives (lobbyists, for example)—or, more realistically at the state and local levels, leaders from professional associations who are lobbying for a policy (and their paid lobbyists if they are fortunate enough to have engaged them)—must have a grasp of knowledge translation. In other words, they must understand how to translate research findings, in context, to various stakeholder audiences. Therefore, step 5—contribute to the health policy development and implementation process—becomes a natural extension of step 4. Together these steps establish the beginning of the policy production and implementation processes.

> Advocacy and lobbying skills are useful throughout many of the EIHP steps but are particularly essential during the integration, decision-making, and development steps—in other words, steps 4 and 5.

Step 4: Integrate the Best Evidence With Issue Expertise and Stakeholder Values and Ethics

As you saw in Table 6.3 in Chapter 6, the issue expertise and stakeholder values and ethics components of the EIHP model are comparable to the clinical expertise and patient values and preferences components of the EBP model, respectively. The details of each component in the EIHP steps have been modified to adapt to the health policy setting. These two components comprise two legs of a three-legged stool that supports the EIHP model, just as their comparable components support the EBP model. The third leg is composed of the best external evidence from global and local sources gleaned during step 2 and critically appraised during step 3 of the EIHP process. That evidence is brought forward and integrated during this step.

Integrating the Best Evidence With Issue Expertise

In the EIHP model, the issue expertise component "acknowledges the professional wisdom of nurses and other point-of-care health professionals and their representative associations" (Loversidge, 2016, p. 29). This component also includes the expertise of other individuals, including consumers and policymakers.

There are three basic categories of issue expertise:

- **Expertise acquired from data collected by a variety of actors who are experts in the issue:** These actors may include representatives of professional associations, representatives of private or independent healthcare organizations, or staff representing government regulatory agencies experienced in and responsible for the implementation of the policy (or type of policy) being discussed.

- **Expertise derived directly from a professional's understanding or experience with a particular health policy issue:** Methods for integrating this type of expertise with evidence include working with professional associations or other bodies to prepare policy briefs or to provide expert testimony at government public hearings (Loversidge, 2016). A standard policy brief generally consists of several pages, but a one-page summary can be very useful and influential when communicating with policymakers. Testimony at public hearings may be provided in writing, orally, or both. (Strategy Tool 8.1, "Guidelines for Preparing and Giving Testimony," and Strategy Tool 8.2, "Guidelines for a One-Page Policy Brief," offer guidance on these topics.)

- **Expertise gleaned from a variety of other available and relevant resources or data related to the policy problem, particularly those related to quality and safety (Loversidge, 2016):** For example, recently, after the manufacturer of a name-brand epinephrine auto-injector exponentially increased its price, one state legislature considered a bill that allowed pharmacists to substitute a generic auto-injector for the name brand, within certain guidelines. In addition to providing lawmakers with a review of the best evidence about the quality of the generic auto-injector compared to the brand-name preparation and expert testimony by representatives from health professions associations and retail pharmacies on the clinical and cost aspects, several stakeholders and advocates compiled data from consumers who were forced to go without the drug because of the cost increase. This provided evidence of potential harm to citizens and additional leverage when it came time for legislators to vote on the bill.

  - This third category of issue expertise might also include that of policymakers themselves. For example, recall the expedited partner therapy (EPT) bill discussed in Chapter 2. Although this accepted evidence-based intervention was legal in most states, enacting a law permitting EPT in a politically conservative state was not a simple task. Fortunately, both primary co-sponsors of the bill were physicians; one served as chair of the committee hearing the bill, and the other served as a committee member. They brought their own issue expertise as both physicians and lawmakers to the process. Without the credibility of their medical expertise and their legislative positions as members of the majority party, the bill may not have passed.

It is particularly important to analyze whether the best evidence—both global and local—aligns with any additional data that has been collected to inform the discussion around policy development. For example, suppose the health policy problem being addressed is a state nurse practice act that restricts advanced practice registered nurse (APRN) practice. In that case, the state APRN association would likely present research synthesized from peer-reviewed journals on the safety and efficacy of APRN practice (including a variety of levels of evidence) combined with the findings of the Institute of Medicine (IOM) "Future of Nursing" report (IOM, 2010) and the Federal Trade Commission report (Gilman & Koslov, 2014), both of which call for the removal of barriers to APRN practice (expert opinion/level VII evidence). These would be considered global sources of evidence. In addition, the state-level association would likely refer to workforce data available from a corresponding national association (global evidence) as well as APRN workforce data collected by the state board of nursing (local evidence). The global and local evidence should be examined to see how they relate and align, or whether one type of evidence disconfirms the other.

Integrating the Best Evidence With Stakeholder Values and Ethics

The EIHP model acknowledges that expertise is represented by divergent perspectives and that stakeholder inclusivity and engagement are essential for gaining momentum for the policy agenda (Loversidge, 2016). Individual stakeholders and the organizations they represent (if relevant) hold core values. *Core values* can be described as "the fundamental beliefs of a person or organization . . . guiding principles [that] dictate behavior and can help people understand the difference between right and wrong" (Core values, n.d.). Core values differ from *ethics*, which are seen as guidelines for human conduct and a uniform system of fundamental moral principles (Ethics, n.d.).

The core values of stakeholders may become apparent as one engages in the work of policymaking. Often they will differ, depending on the category of stakeholder. (Of course, there is no magic laundry list of core values, and stakeholders will certainly demonstrate individual differences within their own categories.) Table 8.1 lists the various categories of stakeholders and how common core values for each category might demonstrate commitment.

TABLE 8.1 Common Core Stakeholder Values and Commitment

Category of Stakeholder	Common Core Values Might Demonstrate as a Commitment To
Lawmakers and policymakers	Government sustainability through the responsible allocation of state financial resources
	Support for certain core programs that will improve the state profile—for example, related to education, access to healthcare, or the reduction of duplication of effort in government
	Manageable change in government policy (incrementalism) versus sweeping change
Regulators	The enforcement of laws and regulations that protect the public over advancing the needs of a profession
	Seeking legislative authority to expand the disciplinary section of a practice act to further protect the public safety
Professional association representatives	Advancing the needs of their professional membership in terms of practice scope/ability to practice at top-of-license or financial interests
	Protecting the needs of consumers served by their professional membership
Citizens	Advocating for a particular cause such as a disease treatment or access to care by offering individual testimony to contribute their personal story to the lawmaking or policymaking process
	Advocating for health policy causes that lean toward conservative or liberal; for example, they might contact their legislators or testify to support third-party payers' rights to require stepped drug therapy to reduce their own co-payment costs (conservative) or to support state Medicaid expansion (liberal)

In addition to core values, stakeholders bring their own understanding of ethics to the policymaking table. The study of ethics is quite complex; however, a brief review of the four basic principles, also known as the *four principles approach* (FPA), follows:

- **Respect for autonomy:** This principle acknowledges a person's right to make choices, hold views, and take actions based on his or her own beliefs and values. It does not, however, reflect a perspective that is individualistic to the extent that it neglects the impact of individual choice on society at large. Nor does it focus excessively on reason over emotion or highlight legal rights over social practice and responsibility. Respect for autonomy involves more than a respectful attitude; it requires respectful action.

- **Nonmaleficence:** This principle relates to one's obligation to abstain from causing harm. In medical ethics, this is a fundamental principle. It's part of the Hippocratic tradition and appears in the maxim, "Above all [or first] do no harm." Nonmaleficence implies a stringent and intentional obligation *not* to inflict harm or evil.

- **Beneficence:** This principle is often confused or combined with nonmaleficence, but it goes further than that. Rather than simply requiring one to abstain from causing harm, this principle requires one to take a helping action to prevent or remove harm and to promote good. This principle results in the making of complicated distinctions in healthcare, where, for example, one might be involved in administering chemotherapy, which causes harm to healthy cells, in an effort to ameliorate a cancer. The distinctions in health policymaking may be similarly complex if a proposed policy might curtail access or freedoms for one population for the greater good. In this case, a greater effort must be made to examine the ethical issues surrounding the policy as a whole.

- **Justice:** This principle, sometimes thought of as fairness, is identified according to perspective and theoretical approach. Approaches to justice have arisen from utilitarian, libertarian, egalitarian, and communitarian theories. More recently, capability and well-being theories have contributed approaches to the principle of justice. An example of distributive justice and fairness in health policy is the allocation of resources for healthcare based on a socially conscious health budget. Fair opportunity, the minimization of discrimination, and the minimization of negative effects are key considerations in applying the principle of justice (Beauchamp & Childress, 2013).

As they undergo efforts to generate a reasonable policy product, all stakeholders must be aware that even the best and most well-intentioned policies have ethical implications. Furthermore, while researchers and clinicians can look to standardized guidelines regarding ethical behavior, there are no current ethical guidelines relating specifically to health policy or health policy research. In fact, the World Health Organization has identified a need to develop a framework for guiding health policy and systems research with regard to ethical considerations.

Although the role of research in health policy is separate from the role of the policymaker, the contexts are essentially the same in that health policy is necessarily influenced by and constructed for real-world contexts (Luyckx, Biller-Andorno, Saxena, & Tran, 2017). Therefore, in integrating the best research with stakeholder values and ethics, stakeholders should discuss whether the policy option being considered as a result of the evidence affects citizen autonomy and avoids harming and indeed does "good" for the target population, and how it might address the issue of justice or fairness.

Stakeholder Analysis

One way to assess stakeholder values and ethics is to perform a stakeholder analysis. This analysis summarizes what is known about those individuals, organizations, or associations.

The stakeholder framework, or model, is based on Mendelow's classic work (1981). This framework/model describes the relationship between an organization and its stakeholders, the organization's need to actualize its goals, and how the relationship between the organization and its stakeholders affects its outputs. It follows, then, that an organization should concentrate its scanning efforts on the stakeholders who have the greatest power over the organization. In the case of policymaking, scanning should concentrate on stakeholders with the greatest power over the policy process. Scanning is a process typically used by an organization to understand its environment. The organization examines external pressures and forces that might affect its function, such as the political environment, progress in legislation aimed at regulating the organization's type of industry, and changes in availability of raw material or emerging technology that might affect how the organization functions (Mendelow, 1981).

Standard methods for stakeholder analysis begin by identifying key stakeholders—the individuals and organizations that have a key stake—

during the policy dialogue. If a policymaker (that is, lawmaker who has agreed to serve as the primary sponsor of the policy in question) has been identified, that person should be considered a key stakeholder. Other stakeholders who might be concerned with various aspects of the policy problem should also be considered.

A second step is to prioritize stakeholders, with the most influential stakeholder at the top. When you do, note details about their stake in the policy dialogue. Also note their means of influence. Ask the following questions:

- Is it political capital?
- Is it financial?
- Is it expertise or credibility?

The analysis should also indicate whether the stakeholder's influence is in a positive or negative direction—that is, will this person or organization be working as an advocate for the policy option or as an opponent?

> It is essential to understand the stakeholders and their motivation, and particularly to appreciate their values and ethics. This will be helpful in the next step of the EIHP model, contributing to the policy development and implementation process.

Table 8.2 contains an example of a stakeholder analysis. The bill analyzed in this stakeholder analysis is a measure sought by the state nurses association to prohibit hospitals from requiring mandated overtime. Mandated overtime is the practice of requiring nurses to work beyond their shift as a condition of continued employment. It can mean an additional partial or whole 12-hour shift after having worked a 12-hour shift. It can also mean a nurse is called back in for a 12-hour shift after having recently finished a 12-hour shift. In many hospitals, nurses who refuse due to exhaustion or the fear of making patient-care errors may suffer the threat of disciplinary or retaliatory action, up to and including termination. In this example, the state nurses association engaged a lawmaker who was willing to sponsor a bill to address this policy problem at the state level. As introduced, the bill included language that would have subjected hospitals that did not comply with the law to penalties. During ongoing dialogue with stakeholders, the paragraph regarding penalties was removed, and the bill moved successfully out of committee and through the full legislative chamber. An examination of the stakeholder analysis will reveal why the state hospital association's request to the legislative sponsor was given serious consideration. If a stakeholder analysis had been completed in anticipation of the bill's introduction, this outcome may have been anticipated.

TABLE 8.2   Example of a Stakeholder Analysis

Stakeholder and Priority Level	Stake and Means of Influence	Direction of Influence
State nurses association	Proposed the legislation as part of a national agenda to eliminate mandated overtime Primary proponent Influences nurses at the state level Gives a low to moderate level of financial and political support to candidates during election cycles	⬆
State hospital association	Primary opponent of the bill as introduced As introduced, hospitals in violation would have been subject to penalties Has significant political capital and credibility at the state level Supports candidates and legislators during election cycles and throughout terms Greater financial capital than the nurses association	⬇
Primary legislative sponsor	Interested in being supportive of organized nursing, minimizing mandated overtime, and moving a bill successfully through the legislative process Enjoys a positive reputation as a member of the majority party and continues to move legislation through to fruition	⬆

RNs and LPNs working in hospitals	Many work in hospitals that mandate OT	
	OT may include being called back in to work an extra shift after having recently completed a 12-hour shift; some nurses report four hours or less at home/sleeping	
	Nurses report exhaustion and are at risk for making errors	
	Refusal may result in disciplinary action or termination	
	Errors or patient harm may result in disciplinary action or termination	
	Have individual voting power	
	Political power is referred through the state nurses association (if they are members)	

The Challenge of Integrating the Best Evidence With Issue Expertise and Stakeholder Characteristics

The most difficult part of successfully integrating best evidence with issue expertise and stakeholder characteristics is the translation of knowledge—that is, research findings—to a form usable to policymakers and other stakeholders. Indeed, the failure to translate research into practice is a consistent finding in both the clinical and the health services (policy) literature (Grimshaw, Eccles, Lavis, Hill, & Squires, 2012).

A number of agencies and organizations in the US and Canada exist to produce research for the purpose of building and/or advancing knowledge about health and transferring that knowledge into policy. These include the following:

- The Agency for Healthcare Research and Quality (2017)
- The Centers for Disease Control and Prevention (2017)
- The National Institutes of Health (n.d.)
- The Canadian Institutes of Health Research (2018)
- The Canadian Foundation for Healthcare Improvement (2018)

Dissemination of research findings is challenging when the audience consists of other researchers and healthcare professionals; it is even more so when the target audience consists of policymakers and lay stakeholders.

There are many challenges in translating knowledge to stakeholders in the policy environment. One of these challenges invites a revisiting of the evidence hierarchy, what constitutes evidence in policymaking, and how evidence is vetted for translation to policymakers and other stakeholders. Nurses and other healthcare professionals are accustomed to seeking a body of evidence, often consisting of single research studies, such as randomized controlled trials, which are closest to the top of the evidence hierarchy. The goal is to find the best most reliable evidence with clear, statistically significant results and internal validity. Evidence is produced by scientists before being filtered and disseminated to policymakers with the intent of changing policy. While this works well when the interventions to be informed by evidence are biomedical or otherwise practice related, the same kind of filtering may be less successful for informing other types of policy discussions. Green, Ottoson, Garcia, and Hiatt (2009) observed the filtering and vetting that occurs in the research-to-practice pipeline and suggested that:

> for . . . most public health interventions . . . the object of interventions is far more diverse in psychological processes, cultural contexts, and socio-economic conditions that may mediate or moderate the relationship between the intervention and the outcome. For these interventions, **context, adaptability, and external validity become as important as experimental control, fidelity of implementation, and internal validity.** (emphasis added; pp. 155–156)

The literature suggests that the best strategies for transferring knowledge involve conveying actionable messages from a body of research knowledge rather than from a single study. Current systematic reviews and other approaches to synthesizing research findings have been suggested as the basic form for translating knowledge to policymakers and other stakeholders. However, some messages can be well-served by providing information from a single study when the study is relevant and placed in context (Lavis et al., 2003).

It is also important to remember that policymakers rely on a number of inputs in addition to research findings to facilitate their decision-making. This point is illustrated by an account of the evolution of nurse practitioners, written in 1984 by Spitzer (as cited in Lavis et al., 2003):

> Decision makers rarely use a regression coefficient to help them solve a particular problem. Rather, over long periods of time, "ideas" enlighten decision makers about a particular issue and how to handle it. For example, it took decades for nurse practitioners to be seen as a viable policy alternative to solve the particular problem of physician shortages in rural and remote areas, and even then most decision makers were probably not aware of the particular studies that demonstrated the safety and cost effectiveness of nurse practitioners. (p. 223)

To reduce the gap between evidence and policy and provide a framework for identifying best practices, current concepts to guide activities related to knowledge translation of research findings have been summarized. These activities are structured around five key questions, originally identified by Lavis and colleagues (2003) and expanded upon by Grimshaw and colleagues (2012):

- **What should be transferred?** The greatest emphasis should be on up-to-date systematic reviews or another type of synthesis of global evidence. Individual studies can also be used, but the results should be interpreted within the context of global evidence before deciding whether it is ready for knowledge translation. Knowledge translators should also identify key messages from the body of evidence, but these depend on the audience. For example, policy briefs are often the most successful means for getting key messages across to policymakers.

- **To whom should research knowledge be transferred?** The answer to this question depends on the purpose of the research and the intended target audience. National or state policymakers, regulatory bodies, and consumers might all have an interest in research, but the relative importance of that research to that target audience varies.

- **By whom should research knowledge be transferred?** The most credible messenger for the target audience should transfer the research. Generally, credibility is built over time. Credible actors are those who have the skill and experience needed to transfer the research knowledge and the time and resources to do so.

- **How should research knowledge be transferred?** Several planned knowledge-translation models exist. Most suggest that success is more likely if an assessment of facilitators and barriers has been conducted. One barrier common across target groups is the sheer volume of research available and its need to be synthesized. A growing body of literature highlights effective strategies for transferring knowledge, including packaging, pushing, and pulling. An example of packaging might be creating an actionable message, while graded entry formats that allow research users to access only the level of detail needed are examples of pushing. Pulling involves conducting activities that create an appetite for research results in the target audience.

- **With what effect should research knowledge be transferred?** The appropriate end point of knowledge translation depends on the target audience and varies by stakeholder group. For policymakers, the desired effect would be that research evidence is considered in policy decision-making, with the recognition that other legitimate policy context factors must also be considered (Grimshaw et al., 2012).

In light of this discussion, let's revisit the stakeholder analysis for the mandatory overtime bill, shown in Table 8.2. A study by Rogers, Hwang, Scott, Aiken, and Dinges (2004) revealed that the risk for error increased when RNs worked shifts longer than 12 hours, worked overtime, or worked more than 40 hours per week. Scott, Rogers, Hwang, and Zhang (2006) studied a random sample of critical care nurses in the US and found that longer work duration increased the risk of errors and near errors in addition to decreasing vigilance. Using a sample of 11,516 RNs, Olds and Clarke (2010) studied the effects of work hours on errors and adverse events. They confirmed prior findings: that an increase in work hours increased the likelihood of errors and adverse events—even when the increase in work hours was voluntary. This is a small selection of the available research on the relationship between work hours and risks to patient safety. A different dialogue might have occurred between the state nurses association, the state hospital association, and the primary legislative sponsor if questions regarding the transfer of research knowledge had been considered and a summary of the available evidence provided. As it happened, they were not. This omission allowed legislators, during the committee hearing, to speculate on the comparability between nurses and food servers working overtime shifts rather than focus on the unique aspects of healthcare versus other service industries.

Step 5: Contribute to the Health Policy Development and Implementation Process

It is virtually impossible to distinguish the end point of step 4, the integration of the best evidence with issue expertise and stakeholder values and ethics, and the beginning of step 5, contributing to the health policy development and implementation process. Recall that the policymaking process is decidedly nonlinear—often spiral or circular. The intersection between these two steps is one of the areas where this is most apparent.

The Health Policy Development Stage

Nurses and other healthcare professionals should take every opportunity to engage in the policy-development process. Whether the policy is being considered in the House or Senate, in a committee or subcommittee, health policymakers must feel the presence of nurses and other healthcare providers.

The same is true with the rulemaking process. Regulatory agency staff often begin rule-drafting long before they publish a public notice for comment. If the regulatory agency convenes a task force of stakeholder interest groups, participation is key. Stakeholders can exert influence from the point of initial dialogue, through rule-drafting, through the comment period, and through the public hearing. If public comment warrants revision, a continuation of dialogue can influence the outcome even at that late point.

During any part of any of these proceedings, it may be appropriate to engage in advocacy and lobbying. Merriam-Webster defines *advocacy* as "the act or process of supporting a cause or proposal" (Advocacy, n.d.). Lobbying is a form of advocacy. Zetter describes lobbying as "the process of seeking to shape the public policy agenda in order to influence government (and its institutions) and the legislative program . . . [and is] the art of political persuasion" (2011, p. 2).

The Internal Revenue Service (2018) distinguishes between two types of lobbying:

- **Direct lobbying:** This refers to "attempts to influence a legislative body through communication with a member or employee of a legislative body, or with a government official who participates in formulating legislation."

- **Grass-roots lobbying:** This describes "attempts to influence legislation by attempting to affect the opinion of the public with respect to the legislation and encouraging the audience to take respect to the legislation."

In either case, lobbying specifically addresses a piece of legislation, whereas advocacy refers to influence focused on a non-legislative policy or cause.

To be fully engaged in the policy-development process, one must advocate and lobby. There's a saying in Washington popularized by Congressman Michael Enzi: "If you're not at the table, you're on the menu." In other words, if you don't make your voice heard, your position is vulnerable, or worse, you've lost control.

Of course, early involvement is better than later—and entering the fray after the process is over is essentially useless. As Zetter observes:

> There are few golden rules in lobbying. One of them, however, is that the earlier you get involved in the process the greater your chance of success. Early involvement also keeps costs down [and] can save the substantial sums involved in retaining a lobbying consultancy to "fire-fight" at a later stage. (2011, p. 3)

Preparing and Giving Testimony

During the course of one's individual, professional, or organizational advocacy or lobbying involvement, there are a variety of methods for communicating one's message. These include providing testimony, preparing and sharing policy briefs, and participating in the policy process in a variety of other ways.

Giving testimony is an opportunity to educate legislators or other policymakers about the impact that proposed legislation or other policy may have, particularly on specific groups of stakeholders. Testimony should be short—typically three to five minutes. (Note that some legislative committees and regulatory agencies issue time guidelines.)

In addition to oral testimony, written testimony is usually required. This will likely need to be provided ahead of a committee meeting or hearing, with hard copies prepared for distribution. In addition, the written testimony may need to be made available for download to an electronic device for policymakers to read during the live oral testimony.

> If you plan to give testimony before a committee, consider attending meetings of that committee beforehand to assess the kinds of questions typically asked.

Strategy Tool 8.1: Guidelines for Preparing and Giving Testimony

Follow these guidelines when preparing and giving testimony (summarized from Loversidge, 2019, and expanded):

- Do your homework. Anticipate questions that might be asked, and practice answering those questions.

- In your written testimony, use lay terminology. Do not use jargon.

- In your written testimony, cite the evidence used. Use a simple citation system; numbers are suggested. Include an appendix with a reference list and access information.

- Bring sufficient copies of your written testimony for the entire committee or policy body, and provide them to the committee clerk or appropriate administrator.

- Rehearse your testimony.

- Arrive early and sign in as required.

- Greet the committee or policy body by its full and correct name.

- Identify yourself and the organization you represent.

- Identify the bill or regulation about which you are testifying by its name and number.

- State your position as for or against the proposed bill or regulation. (If you are an interested party providing expert witness testimony, indicate that.)

- Do not repeat points other speakers ahead of you have made. Instead, if applicable, indicate to the committee that you agree with points made by previous speakers, indicate that your detail points are provided in your written testimony, and urge them to act.

- Do not argue with committee members or members of the policy body, or with persons who have given opposing testimony.

- Begin by providing an overview of your recommendations. Then explain them, point by point.

- In your point-by-point explanation, be clear about which recommendations have been gleaned from evidence.

- Restate your position at the end of the testimony.

- Thank the committee or policy body for the opportunity to speak, and offer to respond to any questions.

- Be clear on protocol. It is common for legislative committee or other policy body protocol to be formal. For example, when a committee member asks a question, the person testifying may be expected to respond first to the committee chair and then to the committee member.

- If legislators ask questions you do not know the answer to, be honest and tell them you will get the answer to them. Follow through after the hearing as quickly as possible.

Strategy Tool 8.2: Guidelines for a One-Page Policy Brief

A one-page policy brief is another helpful policy advocacy communication tool. Effective one-page policy briefs—often called *one-pagers* or *fact sheets* (Short & Milstead, 2019)—are succinct, include only the most relevant information, and summarize major points (Izumi et al., 2010). If an advocate is a representative of an organization, the one-pager should be produced on organization letterhead. Major headings might include the following:

- **A policy statement:** This can be a single sentence that describes the policy action that will be required to address the policy problem.

- **Background:** This section provides contextual perspective and should emphasize any health inequities, disparities, or other issues that help build a persuasive argument. This section should also provide a brief summary of the convincing evidence underpinning the policy action suggestion.

- **Research findings:** This section summarizes the body of evidence. The findings should elaborate on the information provided in the background. It can use numeric or statistical information, graphs, charts, or other visual documents to help summarize essential information.

- **Policy recommendation:** The recommendation in this section should be clear, direct, and relate back to the policy statement section. That is, it should match both the policy problem and the action suggested to address the policy problem. Before writing this section, consider your audience. Who are you addressing with this one-pager? Be certain the policy recommendation is within the jurisdiction of the policymaker with whom you are having the conversation.

- **Contact information:** Provide organizational and/or personal contact information as appropriate here.

Adapted from Izumi et al., 2010.

Building Relationships With Policymakers

Clearly, the role of nurses and other healthcare providers is limited in both lawmaking and rulemaking. In both cases, the ability to make decisions rests with policymakers. Therefore, building relationships and gaining credibility with lawmakers and regulatory agency staff over time is essential. When relationships are established over time, policymakers know who to go to for expert information.

A short list of opportunities to participate in policy development includes the following:

- **Participating on professional organization legislative committees:** Normally, members of the organizational leadership or committee leadership represent the organization at meetings for stakeholders and other interested party meetings. However, members with particular expertise or insight may be asked to join.

- **Volunteering for special-purpose policy task forces or coalitions:** When a policy agenda reveals a special purpose or direction, a task force or coalition may be formed. For example, during the 1980s, in one state that desperately needed a complete nurse practice act revision, a coalition of 41 nursing organizations convened for a period of more than two years to move their policy agenda ahead. This was ultimately successful.

- **Assisting with drafting of bill or rule language:** Some individuals have particular expertise and extraordinary language or writing skills but prefer to work behind the scenes. These people can often be helpful drafting or editing policy language that is offered to bill sponsors or regulatory agencies.

- **Providing expert testimony:** Providing testimony was addressed earlier. Testimony may be provided during public legislative committee hearings at the state or federal levels or before regulatory agencies (both state and federal) that are considering rule changes.

- **Communicating or advocating with policymakers in other ways:** Members of national or state organizations often receive requests to send email messages to their state or congressional representatives about a state or federal bill. The request usually includes information about the policy measure and may even include sample language.

Other methods for communicating with policymakers or legislative aides include the telephone (not ideal, except to establish a relationship) and in-person meetings (preferred). Indeed, you should never refuse a meeting with a legislative aide; these aides are often experts in the policy details in which their legislators are involved.

- **Subscribing to regulatory body electronic notification systems:** It is important to stay informed about any upcoming changes in rules, particularly at the state level. State regulatory agencies have become quite sophisticated with regard to public notification and may have subscription options via email newsletters, Facebook, and Twitter. To find out, conduct an online search for your state regulatory agency or state health department and check its home page. You can also visit the National Council of State Boards of Nursing licensure website at https://www.ncsbn.org/licensure.htm and select "Contact your board of nursing" to locate the website for any board of nursing in the US or US territories.

> State legislature websites may include a link to email a state legislator directly from the site. These are generally configured to ensure only a legislator's constituents can contact him or her. These systems usually require the sender to enter a ZIP code. If the sender's ZIP code falls outside the legislator's district, the sender is likely to receive an error message. That individual will need to contact the legislator's office by another means, such as by phone.

The Implementation Stage

What constitutes the implementation stage depends on whether the policy being discussed is a law, regulation, or other type of policy. If a policy is governmental, implementation is within the purview of the federal, state, or municipal government, depending on the level at which the policy was enacted. Implementation of a new law (or changes to an existing law) generally requires new regulations or revisions to existing regulations. In this case, contribution to the implementation stage can occur during the regulatory rule-making process. If the policy being discussed is organizational, implementation is within the purview of the organization, and organizational norms regarding policy implementation are followed. Regardless of whether the policy being implemented is governmental or organizational, however, contributions can be made during the implementation process.

If the policy is governmental, after related rules are in effect, regulatory agencies may appreciate feedback on their effectiveness. Are the rules reasonable? Do they accomplish what was intended? Was a detail missed or omitted? It is usually a body of key stakeholders who encounter the lived experience of the rules in context after they are promulgated, so any suggestions for future change should be reported to stakeholders' organizations that work most closely with those regulatory agencies.

Summary

This chapter described steps 4 and 5 of the EIHP model. It discussed step 4—integrating the best evidence with issue expertise and stakeholder values and ethics—using the concept of knowledge transfer as a foundation. It addressed the importance of considering stakeholders during the policy development dialogue and introduced a method to analyze stakeholders. It also provided a brief overview of the four ethical principles and their relationship to policy-making. Next, the chapter discussed the essential principles of advocacy and lobbying and strategies to remain vigilant and engage in the health policy process. Finally, it shared thoughts about how nurses and other healthcare providers can contribute to the policy development and implementation processes.

References

Advocacy. (n.d.). In *Merriam-Webster's online dictionary*. Retrieved from https://www.merriam-webster.com/dictionary/advocacy

Agency for Healthcare Research and Quality. (2017). About AHRQ. Retrieved from https://www.ahrq.gov/cpi/about/index.html

Beauchamp, T. L., & Childress, J. F. (2013). *Principles of biomedical ethics* (7th ed.). New York, NY: Oxford University Press USA.

Canadian Foundation for Healthcare Improvement. (2018). About us. Retrieved from https://www.cfhi-fcass.ca/AboutUs.aspx

Canadian Institutes of Health Research. (2018). Home. Retrieved from http://www.cihr-irsc.gc.ca/e/193.html

Centers for Disease Control and Prevention. (2017). CDC organization. Retrieved from https://www.cdc.gov/about/organization/cio.htm

Core values. (n.d.). In *YourDictionary*. Retrieved from http://examples.yourdictionary.com/examples-of-core-values.html

Ethics. (n.d.). In *BusinessDictionary*. Retrieved from http://www.businessdictionary.com/definition/ethics.html

Gilman, D. J., & Koslov, T. I. (2014). Policy perspectives: Competition and the regulation of advanced practice nurses. Federal Trade Commission. Retrieved from https://www.ftc.gov/system/files/documents/reports/policy-perspectives-competition-regulation-advanced-practice-nurses/140307aprnpolicypaper.pdf

Green, L. W., Ottoson, J. M., Garcia, C., & Hiatt, R. A. (2009). Diffusion theory and knowledge dissemination, utilization, and integration in public health. *Annual Review of Public Health, 30*, 151–174. doi:10.1146/annurev.publhealth.031308.100049

Grimshaw, J. M., Eccles, M. P., Lavis, J. N., Hill, S. J., & Squires, J. E. (2012). Knowledge translation of research findings. *Implementation Science, 7*(50). doi:10.1186/1748-5908-7-50

Institute of Medicine. (2010). *The future of nursing: Leading change, advancing health*. Retrieved from http://www.nationalacademies.org/hmd/Reports/2010/The-Future-of-Nursing-Leading-Change-Advancing-Health.aspx

Internal Revenue Service. (2018). "Direct" and "grass roots" lobbying defined. Retrieved from https://www.irs.gov/charities-non-profits/direct-and-grass-roots-lobbying-defined

Izumi, B. T., Schulz, A. J., Israel, B. A., Reyes, A. G., Martin, J., Lichtenstein, R. L., . . . Sand, S. L. (2010). The one-pager: A practical policy advocacy tool for translating community-based participatory research into action. *Progress in Community Health Partnerships, 4*(2), 141–147. doi:10.1353/cpr.0.0114

Lavis, J. N., Robertson, D., Woodside, J. M., McLeod, C., Abelson, J., and the Knowledge Study Transfer Group. (2003). How can research organizations more effectively transfer research knowledge to decision makers? *The Milbank Quarterly, 81*(2), 221–248.

Loversidge, J. M. (2016). An evidence-informed health policy model: Adapting evidence-based practice for nursing education and regulation. *Journal of Nursing Regulation, 7*(2), 27–33. doi:10.1016/S2155-8256(16)31075-4

Loversidge, J. M. (2019). Providing testimony for a regulatory hearing. In J. M. Milstead and N. M. Short (Eds.), *Health policy & politics: A nurse's guide*. (6th ed., pp. 475–476). Burlington, MA: Jones & Bartlett.

Luyckx, V. A., Biller-Andorno, N., Saxena, A., & Tran, N. T. (2017). Health policy and systems research: Towards a better understanding and review of ethical issues. *British Medical Journal of Global Health, 2*(2). doi:10.1136/bmjgh-2017-000314

Mendelow, A. L. (1981). Environmental scanning—the impact of the stakeholder concept. ICIS 1981 Proceedings, paper 20. Retrieved from http://aisel.aisnet.org/icis1981/20

National Institutes of Health. (n.d.). About NIH. Retrieved from https://www.nih.gov/about-nih

Olds, D. M., & Clarke, S. P. (2010). The effect of work hours on adverse events and errors in health care. *Journal of Safety Research, 41*(2), 153–162. doi:10.1016/j.jsr.2010.02.002

Rogers, A. E., Hwang, W. T., Scott, L. D., Aiken, L. H., & Dinges, D. F. (2004). The working hours of hospital staff nurses and patient safety. *Health Affairs, 23*(4), 202–212. doi:10.1377/hlthaff.23.4.202

Scott, L. D., Rogers, A. E., Hwang, W. T., & Zhang, Y. (2006). Effects of critical care nurses' work hours on vigilance and patients' safety. *American Journal of Critical Care, 15*(1), 30–37.

Short, N. M., & Milstead, J. A. (2019). An insider's guide to engaging in policy activities. In J. M. Milstead & N. M. Short (Eds.), *Health policy & politics: A nurse's guide* (6th ed., pp. 215–232). Burlington, MA: Jones & Bartlett.

Zetter, L. (2011). *Lobbying: The art of political persuasion* (3rd ed.). Hampshire, UK: Harriman House Ltd.

"True genius resides in the capacity for evaluation of uncertain, hazardous, and conflicting information."

–Winston Churchill

9

FOLLOW-THROUGH: STEPS 6 AND 7

–JACQUELINE M. LOVERSIDGE, PHD, RNC-AWHC
JOYCE ZURMEHLY, PHD, DNP, RN, NEA-BC, ANEF

KEY CONTENT IN THIS CHAPTER

- Introduction to steps 6 and 7
- Step 6: Frame the policy change for dissemination to the affected parties
- Step 7: Evaluate the effectiveness of the policy change and disseminate findings

Introduction to Steps 6 and 7

Each step of informing health policy with a body of evidence and escorting a policy through the policymaking process is arduous, time-consuming, and challenging. The last two steps of the evidence-informed health policy (EIHP) model are no different. These steps are as follows:

- **Step 6:** Frame the policy change for dissemination to the affected parties
- **Step 7:** Evaluate the effectiveness of the policy change and disseminate findings

This chapter describes these final two steps of the EIHP model.

Step 6: Frame the Policy Change for Dissemination to the Affected Parties

When a new policy is generated—regardless of whether it falls into the category of governmental policy (big P) or organizational policy (little p)—it must be disseminated to end-users, such as citizens, professionals, employees, or some other category. The policy must also be framed in such a way that end-users can understand its intents and requirements.

The inherent difficulties in dissemination are widely discussed in the literature about evidence-based practice (EBP). Even though it's well known that implementing EBP guidelines can lead to improved outcomes, there is often a significant gap between when these guidelines are issued and when they are implemented in organizational policy. Consider campaigns like 100,000 Lives (Baehrend, 2016) and the 5 Million Lives Campaign (Institute for Healthcare Improvement, 2018). By supporting increased adherence to evidence-based guidelines, both have resulted in reducing preventable deaths (Bradley et al., 2009; Wang et al., 2009). And yet, the adoption of national evidence-based guidelines is not universal.

Disseminating policy is likewise difficult—but with one key difference. Whereas the dissemination of an evidence-based guideline may improve the quality of health and healthcare of a population, whether or not that guideline is followed rests in the hands of the healthcare provider or organization. Rarely does a legal standard or organizational consequence require the use of such a guideline. In contrast, if a policy being disseminated is a law or regulation (a big P), then the end-users to whom the policy is being disseminated are required to comply. If they do not, they will face consequences.

For example, suppose a nurse practice act is revised to require a new category of continuing education (CE) and for nurses to confirm they've completed this CE requirement the next time they renew their license. Failure to do so will result in some type of consequence—for example, the nurse's license will not be renewed until the requirement has been met, the nurse may have to pay a fine, and/or the nurse could face a full CE audit. If the nurse's license is not renewed and the nurse attempts to continue to work, he or she will face additional consequences from the state board of nursing. To avoid such a scenario, nurses must be notified of the new requirement before the licensure renewal period in such a way that they understand the requirement and comply. They're not the only ones, however. Regulatory agency staff who will implement and enforce the new policy must also be notified so they can change their work practices accordingly. It is the responsibility of their leadership to actualize this process.

Know Your Audience

Individuals often interpret the same data in different ways depending on the mental model through which they perceive information (Morgan, Fischhoff, Bostrom, & Atman, 2002). Because people have cognitive biases, messages can be perceived differently depending on how they are portrayed. Framing is the art of providing information in perspective and context and is a major element in considering how to approach your audience of end-users.

When framing a policy, the positive aspects of the policy should be made clear, including the rationale. Even if a policy outcome is not what individuals had hoped for or supported, affected parties may be more amenable to new policy standards and more likely to comply if the underlying reason for the policy is clear and rational and the policy will improve healthcare quality or safety in some way—even if indirectly.

When framing a policy for dissemination, it's important to consider audience characteristics. These could include basic characteristics such as the gender, ethnicity, culture, or age of audience members. Or it could be the audience's profession. For example, recall the example of the policy that required additional CE in the previous section. A policy change like this one—likely added to the board of nursing's administrative code—would be written in language that meets the legal standards required by the state's Administrative Procedures Act (APA). Because most nurses—in other words, members of the policy's core audience—do not hold law degrees, this language would likely make it difficult for them to understand the new policy. Therefore, it should be disseminated to this audience in plain language.

When considering the audience that will probably comprise the constituency for a health policy, you should also look at specific characteristics in relationship to the policy. For example:

- Will the policy affect all licensed health professionals or just physicians or nurses or some other group?

- If the policy affects nurses, will it affect all nurses or, say, only APRNs who are prescribers?

If the new policy or organizational rule is based on new evidence-based guidelines, you should also consider the following points:

- Which group of employees will be affected by the policy or rule?

- Does this group of employees have access to an organization-wide information source? How would they find out about the policy or rule?

- Are there other concerns the audience might have that can be anticipated—for example, having the necessary support to carry out the new policy or rule after they have been informed of it and educated or trained to execute it?

> Stakeholders from various audience groups can be helpful when identifying a dissemination strategy because they will have a better understanding of what that audience will need to know and what approach will be most helpful.

Strategies to Improve Dissemination

There are various strategies to improve the dissemination of a policy. One is to identify and engage the assistance of policy champions and opinion leaders:

- **Policy champions:** A *policy champion* is someone who has openly supported the policymaking process and can communicate the new policy to others. Policy champions can be helpful by anticipating social or political pressures related to dissemination and perhaps in overcoming those barriers. If the policy champion is a member of a stakeholder audience, this can be helpful, as the champion will have insider knowledge of any rollout issues. Insider status is not necessary, however, as long as the champion is empathetic to audience issues and concerns.

- **Opinion leaders:** These are people who are recognized by their audience as credible, whether formally or informally. These leaders may be able to successfully disseminate the policy by virtue of their position of credibility. It may be the case that an opinion leader was actively involved in earlier steps of the process—that is, policy development. This is not necessary, however, if he or she understands and supports the policy and can articulate the need for the policy to his or her audience. Within an organization, an example of an opinion leader might be the chief executive officer or a department head. In the case of governmental policy, an opinion leader might be a content expert in a related discipline or a recognized figure such as the surgeon general of the United States (McCormack et al., 2013).

Another strategy to improve policy dissemination is to use one's personal and professional networks. These could be formal networks or informal ones.

- **Formal networks:** These networks involve defined roles and obligations. Examples of formal networks include those between employers and employees and between patients and providers. Employers have an obligation to disseminate a policy if it affects their employees or patients (McCormack et al., 2013), and providers have an obligation to disseminate a policy to affected patients as a part of their professional role.

- **Informal networks:** These networks consist of friends, peers, or family members who share an interest in or will be affected by a policy. An example of disseminating policy through an informal network would be if a healthcare provider told another provider in her friend circle about a policy that could affect them both or told a family member about a policy that would affect him.

Communicating the Policy Change: Who Disseminates and How?

The party responsible for policy dissemination depends on whether the policy originates in government (and if so, which level and which branch) or in an organization (in which case its dissemination is guided by organizational policy).

Methods of policy dissemination by the federal government and by state governments include the following:

- **Federal laws:** These are disseminated to the public through the Library of Congress (LOC). Interested parties can search for federal laws using the LOC website (https://www.loc.gov/law/help/statutes. php) or the website for the US Government Publishing Office (https:// www.gpo.gov/fdsys). One way to search is by category. Codified laws are searched for most often. These are laws passed by Congress that are "general and permanent" and have been compiled into two codes: the Revised Statutes of the United States and the United States Code.

- **Federal regulations:** These are disseminated to the public in the *Federal Register*, the daily journal of the federal government. The *Federal Register* is published every business day by the National Archives and Records Administration's Office of the Federal Register. To access an unofficial version of the *Federal Register*, visit https://www. federalregister.gov/. This version contains the following resources:

  - Federal agency regulations
  - Executive orders
  - Proclamations
  - Other presidential documents
  - Proposed rules and notices of interest to the public

- **State laws:** These laws—generally referred to as *revised code*—are published electronically and can be searched state by state.

> Even if the policy is governmental in nature, there is no reason nongovernmental agencies or groups can't facilitate additional dissemination to stakeholders. What is disseminated, however, must be clearly marked as to its source, and it should be made clear to target audience stakeholders whether the source is official. Private organizations can also choose to disseminate official government documents, which generally reside in the public domain, to members.

- **State regulations:** Like state law, these rules—generally referred to as *administrative code*—are published electronically and can be searched state by state.

Dissemination Examples

A number of successful policy dissemination efforts serve as examples. One of these is a public health policy initiative that began with state-based tobacco control programs instituted in the states of California and Massachusetts (Koh et al., 2005). Both programs involved multilevel interventions to reduce tobacco use rates. Some of the lessons learned from these examples formed the basis for a larger public policy initiative, the Best Practices for Comprehensive Tobacco Control Programs, which was widely disseminated (Fichtenberg & Glantz, 2006).

Another example of successful dissemination is an ongoing policy initiative in Ohio that is part of a larger effort to address the opioid crisis. Recent years have seen a significant increase in the legal prescribing of opioids for pain. This has brought with it several highly negative outcomes. These include an increase in the misuse of prescription opioids and an increase in the use of opioids by persons for whom they were not intended (many of whom eventually transition from opioids to heroin), and an increase in deaths due to opioid overdose. Indeed, between 1999 and 2014, opioid overdose was the cause of death for more than 165,000 people in the US (Dowell, Haegerich, & Chou, 2016).

In response to this crisis, the Centers for Disease Control and Prevention (CDC) published EBP guidelines for prescribing opioids for chronic pain. The guidelines are grouped into three areas of consideration (Dowell et al., 2016):

- The determination of timing to initiate or continue opioids for chronic pain
- Opioid selection, dose, duration, follow-up, and discontinuation of the drug
- The assessment of risk and addressing the harms of opioid use

The CDC disseminated these guidelines in *Morbidity and Mortality Weekly*, the organization's weekly journal, and summarized and disseminated them in a CDC fact sheet. The guidelines were also discussed by other authors in peer-reviewed journal articles and were pushed out to physicians in a special communication of the *Journal of the American Medical Association (JAMA)* Network. Nevertheless, CDC guidelines—even escorted by the credibility of the American Medical Association—constitute little p. Guidelines do not have the force and effect of law, so they remain just that: evidence-based guidelines that *may* be used to change practice.

In 2016, the governor of Ohio determined, as a part of his policy agenda, to act to curb opioid prescribing as a complement to these guidelines and as an adjunct to other state efforts to combat the opioid crisis. The governor asked the medical, nursing, pharmacy, and dental boards to work together to issue uniform regulations for each of their stakeholder groups of licensees. This was a joint effort that was attainable in regulation because legislative intent regarding prescribing—or in the case of the pharmacy board, dispensing—already existed in each board's laws and rules. The respective boards involved relevant stakeholders, filed draft rules, held public hearings, and filed final rules that were consistent across the professions.

The board of nursing's (BON's) rules describing the changes for nurses with prescribing privileges reside in a section that includes the drug formulary and standards of prescribing for advanced practice registered nurses designated as clinical nurse specialists, certified nurse-midwives, or certified nurse practitioners. The rules are clear to a reader experienced in administrative law but could be confusing to most advanced practice nurse stakeholders. For this reason, after filing the final rule, the joint boards developed a plain-language summary, which was posted on each board's website. Although the summary language is not as thorough as the rule language, it was effective in disseminating the main message about the rule change. Table 9.1 compares the language as it appears in the rule (left) with the language in the summary (right). (Note that the rule continues for many paragraphs and includes a much greater level of detail than that shown in Table 9.1.)

TABLE 9.1   Ohio's Acute Pain Opioid Prescribing Rules:
A Comparison of Rule Language and Dissemination Summary

Rule Language (Rule 4723-9-10 OAC*)	New Limits on Prescription Opioids for Acute Pain (Summary)**
(1) Extended-release or long-acting opioid analgesics shall not be prescribed for the treatment of acute pain;	Effective August 31, 2017 . . . new rules for prescribing opioid analgesics for the treatment of acute pain. Please be advised, these rules DO NOT apply to the use of opioids for the treatment of chronic pain.
(2) Before prescribing an opioid analgesic, the nurse shall first consider non-opioid treatment options. If opioid analgesic medications are required as determined by history and physical examination, the prescription should be for the minimum quantity and potency needed to treat the expected duration of pain, with a presumption that a three-day supply or less is frequently sufficient;	In general, the rules limit the prescribing of opioid analgesics for acute pain, as follows:
	1. No more than seven days of opioids can be prescribed for adults.
	2. No more than five days of opioids can be prescribed for minors, and only after the written consent of the parent or guardian is obtained.
(3) In all circumstances where opioid analgesics are prescribed for acute pain:	3. Health care providers may prescribe opioids in excess of the day supply limits only if they provide a specific reason in the patient's medical record.
(a) Except as provided in paragraph (J)(3)(a)(iii) of this rule, the duration of the first opioid analgesic prescription for the treatment of an episode of acute pain shall be:	4. Except as provided for in the rules, the total morphine equivalent dose (MED) of a prescription for acute pain cannot exceed an average of 30 MED per day.
(i) for adults, not more than a seven-day supply with no refills;	5. The new limits do not apply to opioids prescribed for cancer, palliative care, end-of-life/hospice care or medication-assisted treatment for addiction.

*Ohio Administrative Code, 2018

**Joint Ohio Boards, 2017

The state professional association that represents advanced practice nurses and serves as the primary stakeholder organization also facilitated dissemination of the new rule. The association's leadership determined it was essential to get the message out to its membership and posted a news blast, which was distributed to all members via email and appeared on the organization's home page (which was and is available to both members and non-members). Within 24 hours, most APRN prescribers in the state were aware of the change, regardless of whether they had been following the progress of the rule-making process.

Step 7: Evaluate the Effectiveness of the Policy Change and Disseminate Findings

After a policy has been implemented and disseminated, an evaluation of that policy should occur, and the findings of that evaluation disseminated to the audience deemed appropriate, including the public at large if the policy is governmental in nature (Loversidge, 2016). That's what happens in step 7 of the IEHP model. This last step combines evaluation with the dissemination of that evaluation because feedback loops often inform reevaluation, reinspection, and possible revision of a policy.

Policy Evaluation: An Overview

There are two key aspects of evaluation in the context of health policy:

- Evaluation occurs at a different part of the process in EIHP compared to EBP.

- There is more than one way to evaluate policy. That is, policy can be monitored, it can be evaluated, or both.

In the EIHP model, dissemination occurs in two of the steps of the process: step 6 and step 7. The information disseminated in those steps is different, however. In step 6, the health policy change is disseminated to an audience of stakeholders. In step 7, it's the evaluation findings that are disseminated.

The results of an evaluation should reveal whether a policy should continue, whether it needs revision, or whether it should be terminated.

> Recall that policy may be defined as both an entity and a process. A policy subject to evaluation falls into the category of entity. This section refers to the CDC definition of policy because it is simple and includes both governmental and private policy: "Policy [is] a law, regulation, procedure, administrative action, incentive or voluntary practice of governments and other institutions" (CDC, 2017).

Should Health Policy Be Monitored or Evaluated?

People often use the terms *monitoring* and *evaluation* interchangeably, but they have different meanings and implications in the context of policy.

- **Monitoring:** The term *policy monitoring* is commonly used to describe the systematic collection of data to inform stakeholders as to whether a new policy or program is being implemented as designed and according to expectations. In other words, monitoring—which may be conducted by such stakeholders as policymakers, government leaders, managers, and others—is performed to determine whether the program is proceeding as anticipated. Questions that can be answered by the monitoring process include whether policy objectives are being achieved and whether allocated funds are being spent as intended. Data collected to answer these questions include both quantitative and qualitative indicators. Examples include the number of schoolchildren complying with a new mandatory meningococcal vaccination law, the increase in revenue gained by raising licensure renewal fees (quantitative), or how underserved citizens perceive a new category of healthcare worker, called a community healthcare worker, who can help monitor their health status, arrange transportation to primary care visits, and provide other health services (qualitative) (Fretheim, Munabi-Babigumira, Oxman, Lavis, & Lewin, 2009).

> Policy evaluations are not always appreciated or popular among the stakeholders who are required to conduct them or who must make decisions about the future of the policy based on the evaluation (that is, policymakers). This could be because a policy and programs associated with it are controversial or because there is a strong political interest in the policy's success (or failure).

- **Evaluation:** Policy evaluation focuses on the achievement of results. An evaluation is conducted—in particular, an impact evaluation—to determine the association between a particular policy or program and observed changes in outcomes. Policy evaluation typically uses standard evaluation principles and methods and may assess a policy's content, implementation, impact, or all three (CDC, 2013a; Fretheim et al., 2009).

As a first step in the process, you must determine whether a policy should be monitored or evaluated. In the SUPPORT Tools series, mentioned in earlier chapters, Fretheim and colleagues (2009) provide a series of questions that are helpful in parsing this out. If an evaluation is called for, these questions also help you determine how it should be conducted and what should be measured.

1. **Is monitoring necessary?** Whether monitoring is necessary depends on the perceived need. It may also depend on several other factors. One of these is whether an adequate monitoring system is already in place. If not, then you must consider the cost of adding a new monitoring system. If so, be aware that you might need to add new indicators (defined below) to the existing system. Another factor is the likelihood that the findings will be useful. If the findings will not be useful, then the monitoring is not worthwhile.

2. **What should be measured?** What should be measured depends on the policy. This may include any of the following (Fretheim et al., 2009):

   - **Inputs:** These are the information and resources needed to develop and/or implement the policy.

   - **Activities:** These are the actions required to implement the policy.

   - **Outputs:** These are the direct results of the first two measures.

   - **Outcomes:** These are the short-term and intermediate changes that occur as a result of the policy.

   - **Impacts:** These are the long-term changes in indicators.

   - **Indicators:** These are the observable, specific, measurable characteristics of change that demonstrate progress toward the outcome or impact.

Other evaluation questions that help policymakers and other stakeholders understand whether a policy is working, is useful, and has merit include the following (CDC, 2013a):

- Was the policy problem identified correctly?
- Were any important aspects of the policy problem overlooked or omitted?
- Is the policy having the desired effect on the target population or target problem?
- Is there a need for any modifications to the policy as it was designed?
- Should the policy continue?

Additional evaluation questions might focus on the following (Cameron et al., 2011):

- The cost effectiveness of the policy
- What defines the success or failure of the initiative
- What difference the evaluation will make to the policy (that is, what will be done to the policy if it did not meet its objectives)
- What mechanisms need to be established to change or halt the policy based on evaluation results

Regardless of which indicators are measured, factors to consider in determining measures include their validity, acceptability, feasibility, reliability, sensitivity, and predictive validity.

3. **Should an impact evaluation be conducted?** An *impact evaluation* assesses the effects of the implementation of a policy and whether those effects were intended or not (Organisation for Economic Co-operation and Development, 2006). It may be the case that the policy results in unintended consequences or that it affects one indicator but not another. For example, a law allowing family or friends of persons at risk for opioid overdose to keep naloxone (Narcan) on hand is likely to move the indicator that assesses the status of the victim when emergency medical services arrive on the scene (stability of vital signs), but it might not have an impact on the incidence of death from opioid overdose.

4. **How should the impact evaluation be done?** Impact evaluation should be planned well ahead of policy implementation. Otherwise, baseline measures for later comparison may not have been established. The recommended method for impact evaluation is to compare individuals or groups who have been exposed to the policy with those who have not, particularly if groups can be randomized (that is, in a randomized trial). If this is not feasible, a controlled before-and-after evaluation can be conducted. This evaluates a policy to determine the change it has produced since it was implemented by controlling for external influences on outcomes. Interrupted time series evaluation is also a viable choice, during which data is collected at multiple time points. A simple comparison of the value of an indicator before and after may result in misleading findings so is not recommended (CDC, 2013b; Fretheim et al., 2009).

Formative Evaluations Versus Summative Evaluations

An evaluation can occur while a policy-driven program is in process. This is called a *formative evaluation*. If, after you ask whether a program should be monitored or evaluated, the answer is monitored, this constitutes formative evaluation. Monitoring is a type of formative evaluation.

Alternatively, an evaluation can occur after the policy program has been fully implemented. This is called a *summative evaluation*. This type of evaluation seeks to determine whether a program has met its objectives. If so, it looks to identify how the objectives were met. If not, it works to clarify why not.

> Before policy implementation, decisions should be made about data points and collection. That way, evaluation, analysis, and improvement can occur as implementation of the policy unfolds.

There is some tension between uses of formative and summative evaluations related to the pressures and priorities faced by policymakers. In some cases, policymakers receive what data is available to them, and they must simply move the agenda ahead. So, while the evaluation they are in position of doing is technically classified as formative and not in final or summative form, policymakers may feel pressured to act on it as if it were summative. In this type of case, final policy decisions are made based on incomplete information. In other cases, evaluations are clearly commissioned solely for the purpose of providing evidence of impact to rationalize policy decisions that had been made earlier in the process (Cameron et al., 2011); therefore, what appears to be a summative evaluation is made for the purpose of retrospective justification. (Examples of both scenarios appear in the "A Policy Evaluation Example: State Medication Aides" section later in this chapter.)

The CDC Steps for Policy Evaluation

The CDC evaluation framework provides a systematic guide for implementing an evaluation process. Although it was developed for application in public health programs—specifically those related to policies to prevent violence and injury—it is broadly applicable to health policy evaluation. The continuous six-step process is grounded by certain requirements (see Figure 9.1) (CDC, 2013a):

- **Utility:** What audience will receive the evaluation results, and for what purpose?

- **Feasibility:** Are the evaluation procedures practical?

- **Propriety:** Have fairness and ethics been considered in evaluation procedures?

- **Accuracy:** Is the evaluation approach correct, given the needs of stakeholders and the purpose of the evaluation?

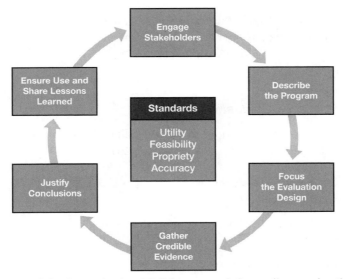

FIGURE 9.1 Steps in the CDC framework for policy evaluation.
(CDC, 2013a)

As shown in Figure 9.1, the steps of the framework are as follows:

1. Engage stakeholders.

2. Describe the program.

3. Focus the evaluation design.

4. Gather credible evidence.

5. Justify conclusions.

6. Ensure use and share lessons learned.

Step 1: Engage Stakeholders

Step 1 of the CDC framework is to engage stakeholders. These might include policy experts, content (subject-matter) experts, people responsible for implementation (for example, staff of regulatory agencies), and evaluation experts. Leadership is essential during this step. In addition, clear expectations should be established during this step so that stakeholders understand the boundaries of their roles.

Step 2: Describe the Program

All stakeholders involved in the evaluation must understand the nature of the policy being evaluated, its intended outcome, and its underlying logic. (Understanding the policy can also be helpful in selecting appropriate indicators and measurement points.)

Step 3: Focus the Evaluation Design

A non-exhaustive list of questions to ask to facilitate the task of focusing the evaluation design include the following (CDC, 2013b):

- What type of policy will be evaluated (a law, a regulation, or an organizational policy)?

- At what level is the policy to be evaluated (local, state, or national/ federal)?

- Was the policy based on evidence?

- Is the policy implementation in progress, or is it fully implemented?

- In what ways will the evaluation be used, and who will constitute its audiences?

Step 3 also involves asking additional questions to evaluate the policy's content. These could include the following (note that this is also a non-exhaustive list; evaluation design depends entirely on the policy that is being evaluated):

- Does the policy clearly articulate the requirements of law, regulation, or another requirement?

- What process formed the foundation for the policy's creation and passage?

- What should inform the impact evaluation?

The evaluation of policy content might focus on the policy's core components, the implementation of those requirements, the evidence on which the policy is based, the roles and responsibilities of stakeholders, or how the content of the policy compares with other similar policies. Policy content should also be evaluated to determine whether it clearly states its purpose, goals, or objectives; whether its requirements are feasible given the resources available; and whether there is a mechanism to monitor implementation. (The latter is often absent from governmental policy unless it is built into law as a sunset provision, discussed in an earlier chapter, or there is a provision requiring evaluation, which usually requires an appropriation.)

> When focusing the evaluation design, consider examining the policy language in its entirety for possible conflicts with other policies, enforcement and compliance requirements, and political and stakeholder influences (CDC, 2013c).

Other considerations during step 3 might include the following:

- **The cost-effectiveness of the policy:** The cost-effectiveness evaluation can be broad. Be aware that this type of economic analysis can be complicated and should be well planned with expert input.

- **General measurement considerations:** These might include population-level data collected over a long period at multiple points in time (CDC, 2013e). For example, short-term outcomes of a law prohibiting texting while driving might be public awareness of the law and an associated decrease in texting while driving with fewer citations. The long-term impacts might be a decrease in vehicular accidents and personal injuries related to texting while driving.

- **Unintended consequences:** Unintended consequences can occur after the implementation of a policy (CDC, 2013d). For example, suppose a decrease in the number of people insured through the marketplace occurs after the deregulation of third-party payers. That would be an unintended consequence. Another example of an unintended consequence would be if a state law required physician oversight for APRN practice, and a psychiatric/mental health nurse practitioner lost access to her patient base when the psychiatrist holding her standard care arrangement retired or left the state without notice.

Step 4: Gather Credible Evidence

Ensure that data collected will be useful in answering evaluation questions (utility) and that the evaluation team will have the time and budget needed to collect the data (feasibility). Also consider whether there are any ethical aspects with regard to data collection—for example, whether privacy or anonymity should be ensured (propriety). Finally, consider the sample size and whether the data will be objective, subjective, internally and externally valid, and reliable (accuracy).

Step 5: Justify Conclusions

When findings become available for analysis, consider the form in which conclusions are presented. The CDC framework (2013d) suggests presenting conclusions in a way that is meaningful and understandable to stakeholders and that interprets the results in a context that considers the evaluation questions and original policy goals. Conclusions must in any case be justified by linking them to the gathered evidence using values or standards that have been agreed upon by the stakeholders. The CDC framework (2013d) also suggests considering alternative explanations for findings, comparing results with other similar evaluations, and considering the influence of possible external factors.

> Data collection and analysis should follow appropriate evaluation methodologies, which are beyond the scope of this text.

Step 6: Ensure Use and Share Lessons Learned

This step is consistent with the final step of EIHP, which encourages the dissemination of evaluation findings. The CDC framework (2013f) encourages the effective communication of evaluation results by using fundamental communication principles. These include the following:

- Knowing your audience

- Framing your message to meet the communication objectives

- Using methods that will best deliver the message

- Considering any restrictions placed on communications by the policy development process so that regulatory procedures are not violated

As discussed earlier with regard to framing the policy for dissemination, the target audience is all-important. Communication objectives and considerations are different depending on whether the message will be delivered to policymakers, evaluators, policy peers, academicians or researchers, stakeholders who will be implementing the policy at the grass-roots level, or the public at large. Table 9.2 contains an adaptation of the CDC's communication suggestions, with the addition of grass-roots stakeholders and the public.

TABLE 9.2 Communicating Evaluation Findings to Various Target Audiences

	Policymakers	Researchers and Other Evaluators	Grass-Roots Stakeholders	Public
Communication Objectives	Ensure the evaluation is credible, meets the objectives of an evaluation, and responds to the policymaker's needs.	Ensure the evaluation work is credible and replicable and meets the objectives of an evaluation.	Ensure the evaluation is credible, meets the objectives of an evaluation, and responds to stakeholder needs for information.	Ensure the evaluation is credible, meets the objectives of an evaluation, and responds to the public's need for general information.
Format Focus	Provide a concise, relatable, easy-to-understand, formatted policy brief. This short brief should include a one-page executive summary or a short Q&A document.	Provide a comprehensive detailed report with the process, methodology, findings, and analysis.	Provide a concise, relatable, easy-to-understand, formatted policy brief or short Q&A document, with availability of full report on request.	Provide a concise, relatable, one-page overview or short Q&A document, with simple graphics where appropriate.
Considerations	Policymakers have little time and are inundated with reports. Ensure the analysis and interpretation is as clear and easy to understand as possible. Frame data in relation to local context, provide real examples to help policymakers relate to findings, and base information on evaluation findings rather than value-based recommendations.	Provide a thorough report. Ensure an absence of bias. Include all background information. Include policy context, demographics, timeline, and resources. Also provide data-interpretation methods, including limitations.	Consider differences in stakeholder groups. Some may appreciate the brevity of the report offered to policymakers; others, such as stakeholders with more scientific backgrounds or interests, may prefer the full evaluation report.	Consider the purpose and objectives of any communication with the public before beginning the evaluation. For example, is the communication intended to raise awareness? Does the public need the information on this policy in order to comply?

Adapted from "Communicating with Policymakers" and "Communicating with Colleagues and Other Evaluators" in CDC, 2013f.

For those involved in conducting policy evaluation, additional sources that provide guidance on best practices in policy evaluation are available. *Public Health Law Research*, published by the Robert Wood Johnson Foundation (RWJF, 2013), describes the most effective ways to conduct public health law evaluation. However, the 2018 update is highly detailed; for a more accessible approach based on the earlier RWJF recommendations, an overview is provided in the article "Measuring Law for Evaluation Research" (Tremper, Thomas, & Wagenaar, 2010). Finally, a policy guidebook published by the United Kingdom and widely known as *The Magenta Book: Guidance for Evaluation,* includes evaluation procedures (HM Treasury, 2011).

A Policy Evaluation Example: State Medication Aides

As discussed, there are myriad challenges associated with executing health policy. One way some policymakers address these challenges is to first create change on a small scale using a pilot program, which can then be evaluated before a full-scale rollout. This often happens when advocacy groups press lawmakers to make significant change, but opposition lobbies make compelling arguments for a smaller-scale compromise.

Ohio launched one such pilot program in the mid-2000s after long-term-care and residential-care facilities lobbied for a category of unlicensed healthcare worker, called a medication aide, to be permitted to administer medications to residents in these facilities (Lanier, 2005). Although nursing organizations resisted this category of worker for some time, shifts in the economy, challenges in the long-term-care environment, and support for the move from legislative leadership forced a change. Nursing organizations were, however, able to secure an amendment requiring a pilot program and subsequent evaluation before widespread rollout by citing evidence related to medication administration safety issues and the potential for medical error (Lanier, 2005).

During the pilot, medication aides underwent BON-approved training programs and were authorized by the BON to administer medications. Although the state authorized the BON to approve as many as 80 nursing homes for participation in the program, only 13 met the criteria established in law and the accompanying regulations. Similarly, although the BON was authorized to approve as many as 40 residential-care facilities, just 12 made the cut.

Lawmakers allowed just 21 months for the pilot study—including rollout, implementation, and evaluation—after which the BON submitted a report on the program findings to the legislature (Ohio Board of Nursing, 2005). This report revealed that no participating facilities were using medication aides for medication-administration duties and that, because of the low participation rate ($n = 0$), there was insufficient data, meaning no analysis, evaluation, or recommendations were possible. Lawmakers extended the pilot in the next state budget bill (Ohio Board of Nursing, 2007), but this extension similarly failed to secure sufficient data to produce a definitive evaluation. Even so, despite the absence of data supporting or refuting the efficacy or safety of the medication aide program, lawmakers made the program permanent.

This example demonstrates several challenges in policy evaluation. One is that politics often trumps data. Even though there was an insufficient body of data for analysis, and despite the BON's transparency with regard to the results of the evaluation, the decision to continue the medication aide program was made for purely political reasons. As a result, the role of government expanded to include a new category of regulated healthcare worker who required delegation and oversight by an RN.

Interestingly, this occurred in spite of the fact that policies that expand the role of government—particularly in the areas of health, education, and poverty—are often controversial. Medicaid expansion and contraction at the federal level and the Affordable Care Act are two examples. In both cases, evaluation data (both financial and programmatic) have provided sufficient information for lawmakers to challenge either the law itself (exemplified in the case of the Affordable Care Act by efforts to repeal or replace the law and by the questions of constitutionality heard by the Supreme Court) or state-level budget-bill support (that is, when states determine to what level they will fund their state contribution to Medicaid).

Summary

This chapter considered the last two steps of the EIHP model. Step 6 consists of framing the policy change for dissemination to the affected parties and communicating the policy change to stakeholders. Important in this step is the question of who disseminates the results of the policy change and how that dissemination occurs. The differences between the dissemination of the outcomes of an EBP change and the outcomes of evidence-informed policymaking are explained. Next, the chapter discussed step 7, which pertains to evaluating the effectiveness of policy change. Practical guidelines for supporting policy evaluation are gleaned from the SUPPORT Tools, which have been established and widely used over the past decade, and the CDC policy evaluation framework.

Coverage of these last two steps brought the discussion of the EIHP model to completion. Both steps are essential to evidence-informed policymaking. Once executed, a policy might be sound and have the potential to produce important outcomes, but it must be successfully communicated to crucial stakeholders and evaluated to determine its success.

References

Baehrend, J. (2016). 100,000 Lives Campaign: Ten years later. Institute for Healthcare Improvement. Retrieved from http://www.ihi.org/communities/blogs/_layouts/15/ihi/community/blog/itemview.aspx?List=7d1126ec-8f63-4a3b-9926-c44ea3036813&ID=268

Bradley, E. H., Nallamothu, B. K., Herrin, J., Ting, H. H., Stern, A. F., Nembhard, I. M., ...Krumholz, H. M. (2009). National efforts to improve door-to-balloon time results from the Door-to-Balloon Alliance. *Journal of the American College of Cardiology, 54*(25), 2423–2429. doi:10.1016/j.jacc.2009.11.003

Cameron, A., Salisbury, C., Lart, R., Stewart, K., Peckham, S., Calnan, M., . . . Thorp, H. (2011). Policy makers' perceptions on the use of evidence from evaluations. *Evidence & Policy, 7*(4), 429–447. doi:10.1332/174426411X603443

Centers for Disease Control and Prevention. (2013a). *Step by step—evaluating violence and injury prevention policies: Brief 1: Overview of policy evaluation.* Retrieved from http://www.cdc.gov/injury/pdfs/policy/Brief%201-a.pdf

Centers for Disease Control and Prevention. (2013b). *Step by step—evaluating violence and injury prevention policies: Brief 2: Planning for policy evaluation.* Retrieved from https://www.cdc.gov/injury/pdfs/policy/Brief%202-a.pdf

Centers for Disease Control and Prevention. (2013c). *Step by step—evaluating violence and injury prevention policies: Brief 4: Evaluating policy implementation.* Retrieved from https://www.cdc.gov/injury/pdfs/policy/Brief%204-a.pdf

Centers for Disease Control and Prevention. (2013d). *Step by step—evaluating violence and injury prevention policies: Brief 5: Evaluating policy impact.* Retrieved from https://www.cdc.gov/injury/pdfs/policy/Brief%205-a.pdf

Centers for Disease Control and Prevention. (2013e). *Step by step—evaluating violence and injury prevention policies: Brief 6: Policy evaluation data considerations.* Retrieved from https://www.cdc.gov/injury/pdfs/policy/Brief%206-a.pdf

Centers for Disease Control and Prevention. (2013f). *Step by step—evaluating violence and injury prevention policies: Brief 7: Applying policy evaluation results.* Retrieved from https://www.cdc.gov/injury/pdfs/policy/Brief%207-a.pdf

Centers for Disease Control and Prevention. (2017). The CDC policy process. Retrieved from https://www.cdc.gov/policy/polaris/policy-cdc-policy-process.html

Dowell, D., Haegerich, T. M., & Chou, R. (2016). CDC guideline for prescribing opioids for chronic pain—United States, 2016. *Morbidity and Mortality Weekly Report, 65*(1), 1–49.

Fichtenberg, C. M., & Glantz, S. A. (2006). Association of the California Tobacco Control Program with declines in cigarette consumption and mortality from heart disease. In K. E. Warner & S. L. Isaacs (Eds.), *Tobacco control policy* (pp. 496–506). San Francisco, CA: Jossey-Bass.

Fretheim, A., Munabi-Babigumira, S., Oxman, A. D., Lavis, J. N., & Lewin, S. (2009). SUPPORT Tools for evidence-informed policymaking in health 6: Using research evidence to address how an option will be implemented. *Health Research Policy and Systems, 7*(Suppl. 1), S6. doi:10.1186/1478-4505-7-S1-S6

HM Treasury. (2011). *The magenta book: Guidance for evaluation.* London, UK: The National Archives. Retrieved from https://assets.publishing.service.gov.uk/government/uploads/system/uploads/attachment_data/file/220542/magenta_book_combined.pdf

Institute for Healthcare Improvement. (2018). Overview: Protecting 5 million lives from harm. Retrieved from http://www.ihi.org/Engage/Initiatives/Completed/5MillionLivesCampaign/Pages/default.aspx

Joint Ohio Boards. (2017). New limits on prescription opioids for acute pain. Retrieved from http://nursing.ohio.gov/PDFS/AdvPractice/New_Limits_on_Prescription_Opioids_for_Acute_Pain-Updated.pdf

Koh, H. K., Judge, C. M., Robbins, H., Celebucki, C. C., Walker, D. K., & Connolly, G. N. (2005). The first decade of the Massachusetts Tobacco Control Program. *Public Health Reports, 120*(5), 482–495.

Lanier, J. (2005). Legislative update: Legislature approved medication aide pilot program. *Ohio Nurses Review, 80*(5), 10–11.

Loversidge, J. M. (2016). An evidence-informed health policy model: Adapting evidence-based practice for nursing education and regulation. *Journal of Nursing Regulation, 7*(2), 27–33. doi:10.1016/S2155-8256(16)31075-4

McCormack, L., Sheridan, S., Lewis, M., Boudewyns, V., Melvin, C. L., Kistler, C., . . . Lohr, K. N. (2013). Communication and dissemination strategies to facilitate the use of health-related evidence. *Evidence Reports/Technology Assessments, 213.* doi:10.23970/AHRQEPCERTA213

Morgan, M. G., Fischhoff, B., Bostrom, A., & Atman, C. J. (2002). *Risk communication: A mental models approach.* Cambridge, UK: Cambridge University Press.

Ohio Administrative Code. (2018). 4723-9-10 OAC formulary; standards of prescribing for advanced practice registered nurses designated as clinical nurse specialists, certified nurse-midwives, or certified nurse practitioners. Retrieved from http://codes.ohio.gov/oac/4723-9-10v1

Ohio Board of Nursing. (2005). Medication aide pilot program planning begins. *Momentum, 3*(4), 13–14. Retrieved from http://www.nursing.ohio.gov/PDFS/Mom/2005FallMom.pdf

Ohio Board of Nursing. (2007). Medication aide pilot program update. *Momentum, 5*(4), 16–19. Retrieved from http://www.nursing.ohio.gov/PDFS/Mom/2007FallMomRev.pdf

Organisation for Economic Co-operation and Development. (2006). Outlines of principles of impact evaluation. Retrieved from http://www.oecd.org/dac/evaluation/dcdndep/37671602.pdf

Robert Wood Johnson Foundation. (2013). *Public health law research*. Retrieved from https://www.rwjf.org/en/library/research/2013/05/public-health-law-research.html

Tremper, C., Thomas, S., & Wagenaar, A. C. (2010). Measuring law for evaluation research. *Evaluation Review, 34*(3), 242–266. doi:10.1177/0193841X10370018

Wang, T. Y., Fonarow, G. C., Hernandez, A. F., Liang, L., Ellrodt, G., Nallamothu, B. K., ...Peterson, E. D. (2009). The dissociation between door-to-balloon time improvement and improvements in other acute myocardial infarction care processes and patient outcomes. *Archives of Internal Medicine, 169*(15), 1411–1419. doi:10.1001/archinternmed.2009.223

"If you find a path with no obstacles, it probably doesn't lead anywhere."

–Frank Clark

10

EVIDENCE-INFORMED HEALTH POLICYMAKING: CHALLENGES AND STRATEGIES

–JOYCE ZURMEHLY, PHD, DNP, RN, NEA-BC, ANEF
JACQUELINE M. LOVERSIDGE, PHD, RNC-AWHC

KEY CONTENT IN THIS CHAPTER

- Challenges with and strategies for advancing the use of evidence by policymakers
- Sweeping reform or incrementalism: developing realistic expectations
- Disagreement from within: establishing ground rules
- Engaging with external stakeholders
- Functioning in complex political systems
- Taking advantage of the window of opportunity

Challenges With and Strategies for Advancing the Use of Evidence by Policymakers

Understanding the policymaking milieu, including its challenges, barriers, and pitfalls, makes it easier to negotiate the process and increases the likelihood of achieving a successful policy outcome.

As discussed, one of the most significant challenges associated with the use of evidence in policymaking pertains to how a body of evidence is presented to policymakers; the form in which it is presented is key. Also essential is how the local significance of the body of evidence is conveyed to policymakers.

As discussed in Chapter 8, "Policy Production: Steps 4 and 5," one strategy you can employ to best present a body of evidence to policymakers is knowledge translation. This strategy involves using succinctly packaged research in ways policymakers find easily accessible and understandable (Grimshaw, Eccles, Lavis, Hill, & Squires, 2012). There are various approaches to knowledge translation:

- **Prepared summary:** This could include summaries of systematic reviews of research or other forms of research syntheses.

- **Policy brief:** A policy brief is a short, succinct document that summarizes key points. Writing policy briefs is discussed in more detail in Chapter 8.

- **Executive summary:** This document—generally no more than three pages—summarizes the main messages of a research report.

- **Graded entry:** This format begins with a summary of the message and a main actionable message—essentially an abstract—on a single page. It then "grades up" to a three-to-four-page summary, followed by a complete project report that should not exceed 25 pages (Grimshaw et al., 2012; Lavis, Permanand, Oxman, Lewin, & Fretheim, 2009).

Another challenge is ensuring policymakers listen to you in their efforts to understand policy options. For example, consider that policymakers sometimes have a need for a specific study to inform a policy, but the time it takes to conduct that study, analyze findings, and translate the findings into policy can be problematic (Crowley, Scott, & Fishbein, 2018; Oliver, Innvar, Lorenc, Woodman, & Thomas, 2014). This often prompts policymakers to seek informal advice, confer with colleagues, or ask trustworthy peers for assistance in locating effective programs to legislate into policy instead (Apollonio & Bero, 2016).

To ensure you are one such colleague or peer, you must intentionally access and continuously work with policymakers in the role of a facilitator (Brown, 2012). This process, whereby policymakers and researchers establish a trusting relationship over time, "may be considered far less difficult than processes associated with a weakly connected researcher attempting to inject un-favored ideas into the policymaking process" (Apollonio & Bero, 2016, p. 463). The value of this kind of researcher-policymaker relationship can be immeasurable in terms of establishing competence and credibility. While these authors (Brown, Appolonio, and Bero) refer specifically to the researcher-policymaker relationship, content experts and stakeholders—who understand and use research but who are not researchers themselves—are advised to form the same kinds of long-term trusting relationships with policymakers.

> Researchers and other policy actors or stakeholders who present the body of evidence must build collaborative relationships with policymakers and be skilled in getting the salient points from the body of evidence across.

Sweeping Reform or Incrementalism: Developing Realistic Expectations

Earlier, we noted that understanding the policymaking milieu increases the likelihood of achieving a successful policy outcome. That means, in part, understanding what policy outcomes might be considered successful. Above all, your definition of success must be one rooted in reality. Enthusiasm for a policy option may give way to unrealistic expectations as to what can be achieved in any single congressional session or state general assembly. But in policymaking environments—whether governmental or organizational— politics often prevail. All this is to say that in policymaking, incremental change occurs more often than sweeping reform, but that this is still a form of success.

> Navigating the policymaking environment sometimes feels like playing the children's game Chutes and Ladders. After moving ahead, you inevitably slide down and lose ground, only to regain it in the next round, and so on. Appreciating that this is a part of the process and learning strategies to overcome barriers and challenges may not make the policymaking "game" as fun as Chutes and Ladders, but it will ease the journey along the road to an enacted health policy.

Incrementalism: The Alternative to Sweeping Reform

Black (n.d.) defines *reform* to mean "to correct, rectify, amend, remodel." Reform is a means by which one improves upon or advances beyond the current state. A reform can be an action of the state (government) directed toward improvements; a reform program is a set of integrated government actions for overall betterment. The idea of sweeping reform connotes visions of far-reaching, comprehensive, broad-brush-stroke change.

When used in a political context, the term *reform* often becomes little more than an attempt to win approval for a program, as when political interest groups use it to advance legislative agendas. The term may come to have deeper meaning relative to the disagreement and struggle it produces between opposing interest groups (Campbell, Donald, Moore, & Frew, 2011).

Still, many policy advocates expect, or at least hope for, policy reform. What occurs more often, however—particularly in government policymaking—is a series of smaller progressive changes over time that may or may not produce the overall desired policy change. This is called *incrementalism* (Hayes, 2017).

Incrementalism is a policy process model first described by Charles Lindblom in the late 1950s. His view of policymaking was that rational decision-making is not possible for most issues for two reasons:

- Stakeholders usually disagree on objectives.

- Policymakers often come to the table with an inadequate knowledge base.

Lindblom described the policymaking process as one in which the multiple groups of participants focused on proposals for policy change that differ only incrementally from the status quo. He purported that the only way significant policy change occurred (if at all) was through a gradual accumulation of smaller changes—a process he called *seriality* (Hayes, 2017).

Incrementalism is understood to have three additional meanings (Hayes, 2017):

- A strategy to make the best possible policy under difficult circumstances, such as when stakeholder values conflict or the information or evidence base to inform a policy is inadequate

- A characteristic of policy due to the bargaining and compromise required during the policymaking process

- A descriptive model that explains how policies are made under usual circumstances and as a strategy for effective policymaking

In combination, these create the impression that incrementalism is an approach to policymaking and suggest there is no workable alternative under normal circumstances.

> While large-scale change may be eventually possible through seriality, the use of seriality as an intentional strategy has been criticized by both politicians and scholars as inadequate to the task.

For stakeholders engaged in the policymaking process, incrementalism in policymaking is a reality. Indeed, nursing and other healthcare professionals see incrementalism at work as they attempt to advance the scope of practice in their professional practice acts to align their ability to practice within the current healthcare environment and in a way consistent with current science.

When a bill is introduced into the legislature, proponents of that bill hope it will be passed in a form that is close to the way it appeared as introduced. However, this is seldom the case. Most bills are amended as they make their way through both houses to the president or governor's desk for signature. During that process, it is a certainty that some compromises will have been reached. In other words, in addition to incrementalism, policies are subject to compromise. Understanding that compromise is part of the policymaking process is essential; so, too, is understanding that achieving even partial success can count as a win.

Compromise and the Myth of Winners Versus Losers

Rooted in the debate about sweeping reform versus incrementalism is the notion that a winner and a loser must be declared based on the outcome of a policymaking effort. In his classic text on society and democracy, Barber (1998) discusses the origins of debate in the legislative branch, once a forum in which parties with opposing interests could feel free to argue an issue and reach compromise. The more contemporary norm employs a popular interest view. This is a less reliable approach because groups in power may make promises but lose support if they cannot keep those promises. They may also lose support if their performance deteriorates as they attempt to maintain control by compromising with power brokers and collecting favors. This can result in a cyclical pattern and ultimately in dissatisfaction within groups (Barber, 1998). It is this competition for control that may result in the declaration of a winner and a loser.

All that being said, compromise should not necessarily be considered a negative. It is possible for every compromise to bring about something of value after sacrifices are parsed out. Little change can occur without some level of compromise, and without some degree of change, the status quo is maintained. Moreover, depending on a stakeholder's level of political capital, total resistance to compromise can be counterproductive. There are two reasons for this:

- Complete resistance to compromise may be reason enough for other, possibly more powerful, stakeholders to disengage from further discussion with the resister. The end effect here may be that negotiations come to a halt, giving the stakeholders with greater political capital an advantage.

- Total resistance is generally perceived to reflect an attitude of disrespect for one's opponent. In the policymaking environment, this will not serve the resisting stakeholder well.

Even after a compromise is reached and a solution is achieved, there will still be stakeholders who are dissatisfied with the outcome. Jacobs and Weaver (2015) noted that policy encounters do not evaporate altogether. After an unsatisfactory exchange or outcome, the stakeholders involved in policy encounters who feel they compromised the most may regroup around opposing stakeholders in an effort to balance their losses. The inference is that a group of stakeholders who feel they have lost ground may target the resulting policy by confronting opposing stakeholder groups and making an immediate attempt to reengage and pursue the hoped-for policy option afresh. Or, they may pause and wait for an opportunity to emerge to regain policymaking momentum.

An Example of Compromise: Advanced Practice Nursing Law

An example of an incremental change in health policy as a result of compromise is found in the nurse practice act in Ohio. Efforts by Ohio advanced practice registered nurses (APRNs) to expand the advanced practice portion of the nurse practice act were made in the 131st General Assembly of the Ohio Legislature. The advanced practice nursing association in that state found a member of the House of Representatives willing to sponsor a House bill that would have made sweeping changes to sections of the nurse practice act had it passed as introduced. The bill contained several significant measures, but most important to APRNs was the elimination of the requirement that APRNs (except for CRNAs) enter into a standard care arrangement (SCA) with one or more collaborating physicians or podiatrists to be able to practice. (An SCA is a written formal guide for planning and evaluating a patient's healthcare that is jointly developed by the APRN and physician or podiatrist.) However, the state medical association opposed elimination of the SCA.

In their testimony, members of the state medical association identified numerous provisions to which they had no objection. These included the following:

- The acceptance of an umbrella term for the four APRN specialties
- Streamlining the licensing and renewal processes
- Removing restrictions on sample medications
- Increasing APRN membership on the board of nursing (BON) from one to two APRNs

Members of the state medical association also made suggestions regarding several provisions. Among these were various compromises with regard to the removal of the SCA. These included the following:

- They called for an increase in the number of APRNs with whom a physician could collaborate from three to five.
- They offered to collaborate with the APRN association.

- They offered to negotiate a compromise on the continuation of reasonable patient care when a physician needs to unexpectedly termi-
  nate an SCA. (At the time, if an SCA was terminated unexpectedly—
  for example because a physician abruptly left the state or died—the
  APRN was unable to continue to practice in the APRN role.)

The medical association was unmoving in its opposition to the elimination
of the SCA and collaboration with a physician, expanded scope of practice,
expanded Schedule II prescribing, expansion of the scope of practice for
a CRNA, and allowing pharmacists to enter into consult agreement with
APRNs.

The medical association's opponent testimony had the effect of stalling the
bill's movement through committee until informal meetings between the two
parties—the advanced practice nursing association and the state medical
association—could be held. Meetings were held over an eight-month period
at the behest of the primary sponsor of the bill. In November of that year, the
medical association wrote a memo to the Ohio Senate, which is where the bill
was being heard by that time, indicating that a position of neutrality had been
reached following a long period of negotiation and compromise. Without that
process and a declaration of neutrality on the part of the medical association,
the bill would not have passed to move APRN nursing ahead in the state, even
incrementally. The bill passed in its 12th version.

The state's Legislative Service Commission produced a document comparing the bill as introduced to the bill in its ninth version. A summary of this
comparison demonstrates the compromises made by proponents of advanced
practice nursing before a final policy solution could be reached. For the sake of
space, Table 10.1 compares 8 of the 15 major topic areas.

TABLE 10.1   Summary of Substitute Bill Comparison Synopsis, H.B. 216

Topic	Bill as Introduced	Substitute Bill Version 9
APRN licensure	Replaces the existing certificate of authority issued by the BON with an APRN license (combined certificate of authority to practice with certificate to prescribe)	Same
Standard care arrangement (SCA)	Eliminates the requirement that an APRN (except CRNAs) enter into an SCA with one or more physicians or podiatrists and practice in accordance with the agreement	Continues the requirement that the APRN enter into an SCA with a collaborating physician or podiatrist and practice in accordance with it. Added provisions in the event the physician or podiatrist terminates the SCA before it expires.
Prescriptive authority	Grants an APRN, including a CRNA, authority to prescribe and furnish most drugs (additional details included)	Same for most APRNs but does not permit CRNAs to prescribe or furnish drugs
Schedule II controlled substances	Eliminates current law provisions that permit an APRN to issue a Schedule II prescription only in certain circumstances or from specified locations	Maintains current law but adds residential care facilities to the locations specified
Drug formulary	Eliminates the requirement that the BON establish a drug formulary specifying types of drugs or devices an APRN is authorized to prescribe	Maintains current law requirement that the BON establish a drug formulary but requires that it be exclusionary

continues

TABLE 10.1   Summary of Substitute Bill Comparison Synopsis, H.B. 216 (cont.)

Topic	Bill as Introduced	Substitute Bill Version 9
Committee on Prescriptive Governance (CPG)	Eliminates the CPG, which consists of four APRNs, four physicians, and two pharmacists	Maintains the CPG but specifies that its membership consist of three APRNs, three physicians, and one pharmacist. Requires all seven to be present to conduct business. The pharmacist is a nonvoting member. In case of a tie, the BON decides the vote.
APRN scope of practice	Defines the practice of nursing as an APRN, with five subparagraphs	No provision
Death certificates	Permits an APRN to certify a cause of death or complete and sign a medical certificate of death	No provision

Summarized from Molnar, 2016.

Disagreement From Within: Establishing Ground Rules

Disagreement or conflict can arise within policymaking advocacy organizations or in workplace environments where internal organizational policymaking occurs. But while dialogue, lively exchange, and a degree of disagreement are encouraged, significant conflict can become a barrier to moving ahead with a policy change. Disagreement or conflict may emerge in many forms and may highlight gaps in processes and ineffective communication (Lipsky, Seeber, & Fincher, 2003).

In her best-selling book *Team of Rivals* (2005), Doris Kearns Goodwin describes how US President Abraham Lincoln staffed his cabinet with individuals who held opposing views to generate more lively dialogue and create a more effective team.

When Disagreement Becomes Damaging

Conflict between individuals with different values and objectives is natural. Moreover, disagreement is needed for growth, progress, and effectiveness (De Clercq, Thongpapanl, & Dimov, 2009; Salas, Shuffler, Thayer, Bedwell, & Lazzara, 2015). You should assume conflict will be part of the policymaking process and prepare for it. Effective communication is one way to cope with conflict. That means ensuring that regular and efficiently managed meetings occur, providing members with time to gain trust, allowing them to feel they have been productive, and addressing any disagreements.

It is essential that disagreements within the ranks of one's own stakeholder group be kept internal. A show of disagreement that extends beyond the limits of the stakeholder group can be perceived as a sign of weakness and provide opposing groups of stakeholders with an opportunity to leverage the dysfunction to their advantage. Disagreement among parties within an organization is usually looked upon unfavorably and is perceived as infighting. *Infighting* is defined as a "prolonged and often bitter dissension or rivalry among members of a group or organization" (Infighting, n.d.).

Infighting

Infighting often occurs when organizations not typically involved in policymaking or that do not have a formal and well-funded structure to engage in policymaking enter the fray. In such organizations, volunteer committees usually do much of the work. In theory this approach is a reasonable way to make progress on a policy agenda. In practice, however, even when the intent is to share work equally among them, a small proportion of the committee members often do most of the work while others remain disengaged. In group-dynamics speak, this is known as *social loafing* (University of Minnesota Libraries, n.d.). This can lead to inefficiencies, resentment toward disengaged members, and a decrease in committee morale. This may become visible not only internally but also to external stakeholders, including policymakers.

In the event of a disagreement or infighting, it is essential for members of a group or organization to *close ranks*. This is defined as "an effort to stay united, especially in order to defend themselves from . . . criticism" (Close ranks, n.d.).

Ground Rules for Meetings

Establishing ground rules for meetings is one way to establish group behavior norms and guide internal team behavior with regard to disagreements. Some ground rules might be procedural in nature, such as rules that dictate that the group start and end on time and all electronic devices must be put on vibrate. Other ground rules are often more abstract—for example, requiring that team members be constructive or respectful. (These may not be helpful if individual members have different perceptions about how those words are defined.) The best ground rules, however, are behavioral. These rules describe specific actions group members should take during meetings and might include the following (Schwarz, 2016):

- **State views and ask genuine questions:** This enables the team to engage in a conversation and appreciate everyone's point of view, minimizes monologues and arguments, and encourages curiosity about differences in viewpoints.

- **Share all relevant information:** This helps the team develop a comprehensive information bank common to all members and facilitates problem-solving and decision-making.

- **Use specific examples and agree on what important words mean:** This ensures team members use the same words, in the same way, to mean the same thing.

- **Explain reasoning and intent:** This enables members to understand other members' reasoning, where others' reasoning might differ, and how conclusions were reached.

- **Focus on interests, not positions:** This moves the team from arguing about solutions to identifying needs to be met to solve a problem, reduces unproductive conflict, and increases the ability to develop solutions to which the whole team is committed.

- **Test assumptions and inferences:** This ensures team decisions are made with valid information rather than private stories, and it eliminates private motives.

- **Jointly design next steps:** This establishes a commitment to moving forward as a team.

- **Discuss un-discussable issues:** This ensures that the team addresses uncomfortable issues that might hinder results and that can be resolved only by the whole team.

While these ground rules are intended to apply to a single team, some of these principles can be adapted for dialogue with external stakeholders with opposing views and agendas. When working with external groups, however, there are significant differences in which rules should be applied and how. These include, but are not limited to, the following:

- Some ideas must remain more closely held.

- Questions and positions should be stated with care and intention so as not to give away closely held information.

- Next steps are not always designed jointly; rather, they are often negotiated.

> As groups gain competency employing these ground rules within their own team, their skill in working across the table with external stakeholders may also improve.

Engaging With External Stakeholders

Policymaking typically involves working with external stakeholder groups who may represent an opposing viewpoint. These opponents may present significant barriers to a policy outcome if a negotiated compromise cannot be reached. To prepare for this eventuality, it is important to understand strategies for engaging external stakeholder groups to advance complex policy agendas.

Engaging with external stakeholders—particularly those who represent the opposition—is particularly challenging. Two possible approaches include the following:

- **Collaboration:** To *collaborate* is to work "jointly with others or together especially in an intellectual endeavor" (Collaborate, n.d.). In collaborative relationships, two or more parties "work jointly towards a common goal" (Collaboration, n.d.). Collaboration between stakeholders is essential during the policymaking process. Note, however, that your ability to collaborate with others who have different agendas and goals depends on a number of factors, including the following (Fischer & Sciarini, 2016):
    - **Common ground:** Working with other stakeholders who might have opposing goals requires identifying shared opinions or interests. For example, both advanced practice nursing

association and medical association representatives share an interest in patient safety.

- **Perceived power:** The perceived power of another stakeholder group may depend on how powerful one perceives one's own group to be, or it could be a product of how much political capital that external group has with other stakeholders, such as other external groups and policymakers.

- **Cooperation:** Cooperative behavior is different from collaborative behavior. It requires patience, persistence, and a degree of confidence in one's objectives.

Interestingly, although cooperative behavior has been a subject of study by social, biological, and psychological scientists, much of our understanding of cooperative behavior derives from game theory. In particular, Robert Axelrod's (2006) research on cooperation focused on exploring interactions between group members who pursued their own self-interest. In his research, Axelrod used the classic computer-simulation game Prisoner's Dilemma (PD), which asks the question, "When should a person cooperate, and when should a person be selfish, in an ongoing interaction with another person?" (p. vii). There are numerous versions of PD, but the most powerful one is a simple mathematical strategy called *Tit for Tat* (TFT). The TFT strategy instructs players move-by-move in the game. On the first move, and the first meeting with the opponent, the strategy is to cooperate. After that, the player copies whatever the other player did on his or her previous move.

TFT has three characteristics (Axelrod, 1997; Axelrod, 2006; Dugatkin, 1998):

- **It is nice:** TFT always begins by cooperating, so it is nice. Niceness allows for the serial initiation and continuation of cooperative exchanges.

- **It allows for retaliation:** This applies if the opponent defects in the exchange—in other words, fails to cooperate on the next move. Retaliation is protective and guards against cheating on the part of the competitor.

- **It is forgiving:** TFT recalls only the last move. This prevents the possibility of continued defections on the basis of a single move and considers that a player may have erred in the most recent move.

Of course, unlike with a computer-simulated game, there is no formulaic method for engaging with external stakeholders. However, although PD and TFT are games that use mathematical modeling, the fact that those models have been applied successfully in exchanges of human behavior are compelling. TFT in particular provides some guidance in working with external stakeholders with whom you are likely to interact again but who have different policy agendas and goals from yours. It follows the basic principles encouraged by President Lincoln in his cabinet: Engage in lively dialogue, debate, and disagree, but then shake hands and move on.

> Both collaboration and cooperation can be useful in establishing the foundations of relationships with policymakers and other stakeholders. These working relationships are essential for success in policymaking—particularly over the long term.

Functioning in Complex Political Systems

The policymaking environment is complex; this is self-evident. The structure and function of government bodies—from Capitol Hill to state capitols to municipal government—make the policymaking environment difficult to navigate under the best of circumstances. (The structure and function of healthcare organizations in which nurses and other healthcare providers work can be just as multifaceted and just as political.) Moreover, even when one understands how a bill becomes a law, which chambers have what functions, how bills are assigned to committee, and the role of a primary sponsor and committee chair, this can be trumped by partisan politics or a disagreement with an opposing stakeholder.

Navigating political complexities takes time, patience, and experience. So, why do nurses and other healthcare providers persist in working to advance good, evidence-informed health policy (EIHP)? The answer is embedded in what we do and who we are. Professionals who are in the business of healthcare are generally passionate about what they do and have a strong motivation to make a difference. Even when the barriers seem insurmountable, healthcare professionals have the background, the story, and the skills to gather the body of evidence to make strong arguments for advancing sound EIHP.

To take part in a policy agenda resulting in the execution of EIHP, you must engage in the steps of policymaking and dive head-long into the complexities of the policymaking system. To avoid feeling overwhelmed by the process, you must understand and appreciate system complexities. Among these are the partisan politics and leadership structures, and the importance of costs on policy outcomes, both addressed in Chapter 5. Because of the nature of complexity, mentors in policymaking can play an essential role.

Mentors in Policymaking

Seeking the support of mentors is useful for navigating the complexity of the policymaking system. Having a mentor offers the following advantages:

- A mentor can guide individuals who are new to a professional or trade organization's legislative committee become productive members of those committees.

- Mentors can help novices learn to think through strategy; talk with policymakers; prepare policy briefs, talking points, fact sheets, or testimony; and navigate the policymaking system.

- Having a mentor on hand at your first legislative or congressional committee hearing makes for a much more comfortable and productive experience.

- A mentor can help coach you on how to package and express your policy message (sometimes called the *spin*).

If an organization has the financial resources to employ a lobbying firm, a paid lobbyist can serve in this role, in part. Although working with a contract lobbyist is different from developing a mentor relationship with a professional colleague, a lobbyist's expert understanding of the political environment, the players, and the process can be incredibly illuminating.

Taking Advantage of the Window of Opportunity

Recall the discussion of the Kingdon streams model (1995) in Chapter 5, "Policymaking Processes and Models." That model identified three types of processes in policy formulation, called *streams:* the problem stream, the policy stream, and the politics stream. When these three streams converge, it is said that the policy window opens.

All too often stakeholders new to policymaking fail to account for all three streams. For example, they might identify a policy problem (problem stream) and design a sound policy solution (policy stream) but fail to account for the political environment (political stream), which accounts for factors such as election and budget cycles, the national or state mood, and the sense of special interest stakeholder groups. Or they might identify a policy problem and account for the political environment but fail to design a sound policy solution. But without the alignment of the three streams—problem, policy, and politics—the policy window remains closed.

To avoid feeling frustrated or overwhelmed by the policy process, it's imperative that you assess the big picture and develop a plan that covers contingencies related to all three streams. Failure to do so is sure to result in chaos within the ranks and the derailment of your policy agenda. Once that happens, the window of opportunity closes and may never open again.

Summary

Of particular importance is how evidence is gathered, synthesized, packaged, and shared with policymakers so that it is relevant and usable and will have a positive impact on the policy outcome. Strategies for using evidence to advance EIHP are found throughout this text. At the end of the day, what nurses and other healthcare providers, policymakers, other stakeholders, and citizens hope for is advancement of the best possible health policy, informed by a sound body of evidence.

This chapter discussed challenges and facilitators to advancing the use of evidence by policymakers. Included among the challenges are the difficulties encountered in getting current and relevant evidence into the hands of policymakers in such a way that it is understandable and usable. Strategies come from the science of knowledge translation and include packaging approaches such as policy briefs and summaries, as well as the development of communication pathways.

The benefits of developing long-term relationships with policymakers rather than short-term single-purpose relationships were addressed by this chapter. It also discussed the challenges associated with expectations and the fact that much of policymaking is incremental. Learning to develop realistic expectations and perfecting the art of compromise are essential in policymaking. While many see compromise as a barrier, it's simply part of the process.

This chapter also examined one of the most challenging issues in working with internal stakeholder groups: establishing ground rules to ensure the group closes ranks to prevent external stakeholders from taking advantage of perceived group weakness. That discussion segued into a conversation about engaging with external stakeholders. The chapter drew from collaboration and cooperation theory to address strategies for working with stakeholders who have a different policymaking agenda and goals. Finally, the chapter addressed some additional complexities of the policymaking process, presented strategies and tools to manage those complexities, and reaffirmed the importance of the use of evidence in health policymaking.

References

Apollonio, D. E., & Bero, L. A. (2016). Challenges to generating evidence-informed policy and the role of systematic reviews and (perceived) conflicts of interest. *Journal of Communication in Healthcare, 9*(2), 135–141. doi:10.1080/17538068.2016.1182784

Axelrod, R. (1997). *The complexity of cooperation.* Princeton, NJ: Princeton University Press.

Axelrod, R. (2006). *The evolution of cooperation* (Revised ed.). New York, NY: Basic Books.

Barber, Benjamin. (1998). *A place for us: How to make a society civil and democracy strong.* New York, NY: Hill and Wang.

Black, H. C. (n.d.). Reform. In *Black's law dictionary* (2nd ed.). Retrieved from https://thelawdictionary.org/reform/

Brown, C. (2012). The 'policy-preferences model': A new perspective on how researchers can facilitate the take-up of evidence by educational policy makers. *Evidence & Policy, 8*(4), 455–472. doi:10.1332/174426412X660106

Campbell, D., Donald, B., Moore, G., & Frew, D. (2011). Evidence check: Knowledge brokering to commission research reviews for policy. *Evidence & Policy, 7*(1), 91–107. doi:10.1332/174426411X553034

Close ranks. (n.d.). In *Cambridge dictionary.* Retrieved from https://dictionary.cambridge.org/us/dictionary/english/close-ranks

Collaborate. (n.d.). In *Merriam-Webster's online dictionary.* Retrieved from https://www.merriam-webster.com/dictionary/collaborate

Collaboration. (n.d.). In *BusinessDictionary.* Retrieved from http://www.businessdictionary.com/definition/collaboration.html

Crowley, M., Scott, J. T. B., & Fishbein, D. (2018). Translating prevention research for evidence-based policymaking: Results from the Research-to-Policy Collaboration pilot. *Prevention Science, 19*(2), 260–270. doi:10.1007/s11121-017-0833-x

De Clercq, D., Thongpapanl, N., & Dimov, D. (2009). When good conflict gets better and bad conflict becomes worse: The role of social capital in the conflict–innovation relationship. *Journal of the Academy of Marketing Science, 37*, 283–297. doi:10.1007/s11747-008-0122-0

Dugatkin, L. A. (1998). Game theory and cooperation. In L. A. Dugatkin & H. K. Reeve (Eds.), *Game theory and animal behavior* (pp. 38–63). Oxford, UK: Oxford University Press.

Fischer, M., & Sciarini, P. (2016). Drivers of collaboration in political decision making: A cross-sector perspective. *The Journal of Politics, 78*(1), 63–74.

Goodwin, D. K. (2005). *Team of rivals: The political genius of Abraham Lincoln.* New York, NY: Simon & Schuster.

Grimshaw, J. M., Eccles, M. P., Lavis, J. N., Hill, S. J., & Squires, J. E. (2012). Knowledge translation of research findings. *Implementation Science, 7*(50) doi:10.1186/1748-5908-7-50

Hayes, M. (2017). Incrementalism and public policy-making. *Oxford research encyclopedias.* doi:10.1093/acrefore/9780190228637.013.133

Infighting. (n.d.). In *Merriam-Webster's online dictionary.* Retrieved from https://www.merriam-webster.com/dictionary/infighting

Jacobs, A. M., & Weaver, R. K. (2015). When policies undo themselves: Self-undermining feedback as a source of policy change. *Governance, 28*(4), 441–457. doi:10.1111/gove.12101

Kingdon, J. W. (1995). *Agendas, alternatives, and public policies* (2nd ed.). Harlow, UK: Longman.

Lavis, J. N., Permanand, G., Oxman, A. D., Lewin, S., & Fretheim, A. (2009). SUPPORT tools for evidence-informed health policymaking (STP) 13: Preparing and using policy briefs to support evidence-informed policymaking. *Health Research Policy and Systems, 7*(Suppl. 1), S13. doi:10:1186/1478-4505-7-S1-S13

Lipsky, D. B., Seeber, R. L., & Fincher, R. (2003). *Emerging systems for managing workplace conflict: Lessons from American corporations for managers and dispute resolution professionals.* San Francisco, CA: Jossey-Bass.

Molnar, E. (2016). Ohio Legislative Service Commission sub bill comparative synopsis, HB 216. Retrieved from https://www.legislature.ohio.gov/download?key=5333&format=pdf

Oliver, K., Innvar, S., Lorenc, T., Woodman, J., & Thomas, J. (2014). A systematic review of barriers to and facilitators of the use of evidence by policymakers. *BMC Health Services Research, 14*(1), 2. doi:10.1186/1472-6963-14-2

Salas, E., Shuffler, M. L., Thayer, A. L., Bedwell, W. L., & Lazzara, E. H. (2015). Understanding and improving teamwork in organizations: A scientifically based practical guide. *Human Resource Management, 54*(4), 599–622. doi:10.1002/hrm.21628

Schwarz, R. (2016, June 15). 8 ground rules for great meetings. *Harvard Business Review.* Retrieved from https://hbr.org/2016/06/8-ground-rules-for-great-meetings

University of Minnesota Libraries. (n.d.). Group dynamics. Retrieved from http://open.lib.umn.edu/principlesmanagement/chapter/13-3-group-dynamics/

A

RESOURCES

This appendix includes a number of resources helpful to
individuals who seek to inform themselves on evidence-based
policymaking. It is organized into sections focused on the US
federal government (including governmental and nongovernmental sources), global resources including those from
the World Health Organization (WHO), and a resource for
organizational health policymaking. The appendix ends with
two general resources for practice: a "Research Insights"
brief from Academy Health that provides a way to approach
rapid evidence review specific to health policy and practice,
and an overview of "SUPPORT Tools for Evidence-Informed
Health Policymaking (STP)."

United States Federal Government Resources

USA.gov

https://www.usa.gov/
USA.gov serves as an entry point for information about the US federal government. It includes links to government services and information by topic, such as the following:

- About the US
- Benefits, Grants, Loans
- Consumer Issues
- Disability Services
- Disasters and Emergencies
- Earth and the Environment
- Education
- Government Agencies and Elected Officials
- Health
- Housing
- Jobs and Unemployment
- Laws and Legal Issues
- Military and Veterans
- Money and Credit
- Small Business
- Travel and Immigration
- Voting and Elections

Of particular note here is the Government Agencies and Elected Officials section (https://www.usa.gov/agencies), which offers access to the following resources:

- A-Z Index of US Government Agencies
- About the US
- Branches of Government
- Budget of the US Government
- Buying from the US Government
- Contact Elected Officials
- Contact Government by Topic
- Forms, by Agency
- State, Local, and Tribal Governments

The White House

https://www.whitehouse.gov/
This site enables you to sign up for email updates, view live-streamed events, and learn about the building itself as well as past presidents and first ladies. The site also offers a description of the three branches of government and has the following links:

- Elections and Voting

- Federal Agencies & Commissions

- State & Local Government

US Senate

https://www.senate.gov/
This site contains the following links:

- **Senators:** Clicking this link offers access to contact information for current senators, information about current Senate leadership, and information about former senators. This link also offers access to information about qualifications and terms of service, facts and milestones, and states.

- **Committees:** This link has information about committee membership and assignments, hearings and meetings, and history.

- **Legislation and Records:** Click this link to access information about bills (by number), congressional votes, and active legislation. You can also click this link to access resources that track recent floor activity, including the Congressional Record (a verbatim account of the Senate's proceedings), the Daily Digest (which summarizes the day's floor and committee actions and lists measures scheduled for action during the next meeting), and Roll Call Votes (which lists the most recent session at the top).

US House of Representatives

https://www.house.gov/
This site's main page, which lists the current number and session of Congress, enables you to quickly look up your representative (via ZIP code). You can also quickly ascertain whether the House is currently in session. The main page also offers the following links:

- **Representatives:** Click this link to access a directory of representatives searchable by state and district or by last name.

- **Leadership:** To identify the current House leadership—including the speaker of the House and leaders of the current majority and minority parties—click this link.

- **Committees:** This link directs you to a page that lists all permanent House committees, with links to each committee's page.

- **Legislative Activity:** This link opens a page that contains a calendar that shows district work periods, days in session, federal holidays, and events. It also contains a list of events scheduled for the day (if applicable). Finally, the page offers the following links:

  - House Floor Proceedings

  - House Committee Live Video Streams

  - Daily Digest

  - House Calendar

  - Federal Holidays

- **The House Explained:** For descriptions of the branches of government, the legislative process, officers and organizations, and so on, click this link.

Office of the Federal Register

https://www.archives.gov/federal-register
The Office of the Federal Register is an office of the US government. It is part of the National Archives and Records Administration. The office publishes the *Federal Register*, the Code of Federal Regulations, public papers of US presidents, and the US Statutes at Large, among other federal documents.

Two links on the office's main page deserve additional description:

- **Federal Register in XML:** The US Government Publishing Office (GPO) makes certain collections of information available in bulk in XML, a machine-readable format, via a bulk data repository. The *Federal Register* in XML is such a collection and is available via the home page for the Office of the Federal Register.

- **Electronic CFR:** Called the e-CFR, this is an unofficial edition of the Code of Federal Regulations. It is an editorial compilation of CFR material, as well as amendments from the *Federal Register*, and is produced by the National Archives and Records Administration's Office of the Federal Register and the GPO. The e-CFR is updated daily and is linked to the *Federal Register* home page.

In addition to these, the home page for the Office of the Federal Register contains the following useful links:

- Executive Orders

- Find a Document

- Hot Off the Presses

- Public Laws

- Today's Federal Register

The Rules & Regulations section of the page offers links to the daily and annual CFR, and the From the White House section provides direct access to various presidential documents, including executive orders. Finally, the Public Workshops section offers information about upcoming public workshops (if applicable).

"Overview of CDC's Policy Process"

https://www.cdc.gov/policy/analysis/process/docs/cdcpolicyprocess.pdf
The Centers for Disease Control and Prevention (CDC) is a federal government agency under the purview of the US Department of Health and Human Services. This 2012 document from the CDC summarizes the domains of the CDC policy process. Although its primary audience is public health practitioners, its policy domains and processes are widely applicable to health policymaking.

US-Focused Nongovernmental Resources

"Working With Congress: A Scientist's Guide to Policy"

https://mcmprodaaas.s3.amazonaws.com/s3fs-public/AAAS_Working_with_Congress.pdf
This document, written by Kasey Shewey White and Joanne P. Carney and published in 2011 by the American Association for the Advancement of Science, was developed to facilitate communication between scientists and policymakers. Its primary audience is scientists who conduct research that informs policy. Chapters 1 and 2 provide background information on the structure of Congress and the legislative process, and Chapter 3 includes communication strategies and rules for working with congressional lawmakers.

GovTrack.us

https://www.govtrack.us/
While not a direct vehicle of the federal government, GovTrack.us publishes reliable information about the status of federal legislation, the women and men who serve in Congress, and voting records, and includes original research on bills and votes.

Of particular note on the GovTrack main page is the Congress menu. This menu contains the following useful options:

- **Members of Congress:** Select this option to access a page that enables you to locate your representatives, view a map of all congressional districts, see all members of Congress, and even find information about former members of Congress.

- **Bills and Resolutions:** This option enables you to access information about upcoming and trending bills and resolutions, to locate information about a specific bill, and to sign up to receive alerts about major legislative activity, upcoming legislation, new laws, new bills and resolutions, and more.

- **Voting Records:** Choose this option to track voting records by bill or resolution. You can also choose to receive an email when Congress votes on a bill or other matter.

- **Committees:** To track upcoming congressional committee meetings, click this link.

Global Resources

WHO Handbook for Guideline Development (2nd Ed.)

http://apps.who.int/medicinedocs/documents/s22083en/s22083en.pdf
The World Health Organization (WHO) produces and disseminates guidelines useful for informing public health policy on a global scale. These guidelines are especially useful for low- and middle-income nations. This handbook, prepared by Susan L. Norris in 2014, outlines how the WHO develops these guidelines. A WHO guideline is a document that contains recommendations for either clinical practice or public health policy and has been developed by the WHO. The guidelines provide general stepwise guidance for guideline development and include the important aspects of equity, human rights, gender, and social determinants of health considerations in guideline generation. The guidelines are based on the use of scientific evidence and acknowledge that the science that drives how evidence is identified, synthesized, and translated into recommendations is continuously evolving.

GRADE Working Group

http://www.gradeworkinggroup.org/
In 2000, the Grading of Recommendations Assessment, Development and Evaluation (GRADE) working group formed to address shortcomings in healthcare grading systems. Since then, with input from many international organizations (including the WHO), the GRADE working group has developed an approach to assess the quality (or certainty) of evidence and strength of recommendations, which has since become the de facto standard for both clinicians and policymakers. Today, there are nine GRADE centers and three GRADE networks worldwide. Additionally, more than 100 organizations representing 19 countries from around the world have endorsed or use GRADE (GRADE, n.d.).

GRADE guidelines facilitate health policy decision-making by facilitating judg-ments about research study quality or certainty. This enables policymakers to judge the potential benefits versus harms based on the strength of recommen-dations; confidence ratings are high, moderate, low, or very low (Alexander et al., 2016; Guyatt et al., 2011; Guyatt et al., 2008; Oxman, Lavis, & Fretheim, 2007; Schünemann, Fretheim, Oxman, & WHO Advisory Committee on Health Research, 2006).

The GRADE working group includes a Getting Started section, which of-fers links to a series of articles in *BMJ* from 2008, introductory lectures, the GRADEpro guideline-development tool, and GRADE events and workshops worldwide. Links to publications—both quick and in-depth reads—are also available.

"Stakeholder Analysis Guidelines"

http://www.who.int/workforcealliance/knowledge/toolkit/33.pdf
This document was authored by Kammi Schmeer and published in 2000 by the Health Sector Reform Initiative in cooperation with the WHO. It is one section of a larger document called the *Policy Toolkit for Strengthening Health Sector Reform*. Although it is older, its guidelines still stand, and the principles upon which the guidelines are based are applicable across a broad range of policymaking initiatives.

"Engaging With Academics: How to Further Strengthen Open Policymaking"

https://assets.publishing.service.gov.uk/government/uploads/system/uploads/attachment_data/file/283129/13-581-engaging-with-academics-open-policy-making.pdf
This practical guide, issued in 2013 by the UK Government Office for Science, is aimed at policymakers who have a legislative focus in science-, technology-, or engineering-related areas but is also intended to be of use to any policy-maker or person in government who works with evidence. It is a concise and constructive guidebook, complete with case studies, and is designed to pro-mote engagement between policymakers and academics.

"A Guide to Engaging With Government for Academics"

https://assets.publishing.service.gov.uk/government/uploads/system/uploads/
attachment_data/file/283118/11-1360-guide-engaging-with-government-for-
academics.pdf
A two-page document, "A Guide to Engaging with Government for
Academics," is also available for government officials and policymakers. It
includes links to resources such as the UK Government Office for Science; the
Department for Business, Energy & Industrial Strategy; the Office of the Prime
Minister; and others. While this document is UK-specific, the "Ask Yourself
Some Questions" section is applicable to evidence-informed policymaking
regardless of place of origin.

Canadian Foundation for Healthcare Improvement Organizational Assessment Tool

https://www.cfhi-fcass.ca/PublicationsAndResources/cfhi-self-assessment-tool
This tool was created in 2014 by the Canadian Foundation for Healthcare
Improvement (CFHI) to assist healthcare organizations in assessing their readiness and capacity to undertake improvement initiatives. The CFHI's Healthcare Improvement Model includes six aspects, one of which is promoting
evidence-informed decision-making.

General Resources for Practice

"Research Insights: Rapid Evidence Reviews for Health Policy and Practice"

https://www.academyhealth.org/sites/default/files/rapid_evidence_reviews_
brief_january_2016.pdf
AcademyHealth "works to improve health and the performance of the health
system by supporting the production and use of evidence to inform policy
and practice" (AcademyHealth, 2018). This 2016 brief provides an overview
of different approaches for conducting rapid reviews of evidence. Although
nurses and other healthcare providers are most familiar with the types of rapid
reviews used in clinical decision-making, such as rapid critical appraisal, the
focus here is on evidence that informs health policymaking. The terms *brief*

review, rapid review, evidence summary, rapid review, rapid evidence assessment, and *rapid synthesis* are differentiated, rationale for their use is provided, and sources in the literature are identified.

"SUPPORT Tools for Evidence-Informed Health Policymaking (STP)"

https://health-policy-systems.biomedcentral.com/articles/supplements/volume-7-supplement-1
In 2009, *Health Research Policy and Systems* devoted a supplemental issue to a series of articles designed to support those involved in using evidence to support health policymaking. This series, known as "SUPPORT Tools for Evidence-Informed Health Policymaking (STP)," is as relevant today as it was when it was written.

The series was prepared as part of the SUPPORT project, underwritten by the European Commission's 6th Framework INCO programme. The series addressed four broad areas (Oxman & Hanney, 2009, p. 1):

- Supporting evidence-informed policymaking
- Identifying needs for research evidence in relation to three steps in policymaking processes: problem clarification, options framing, and implementation planning
- Finding and assessing systematic reviews and other types of evidence to inform these steps
- Going from research evidence to decisions

The introduction and series of "18 SUPPORT Tools" articles are in the public domain and can be downloaded in PDF form from https://health-policy-systems.biomedcentral.com/articles/supplements/volume-7-supplement-1. All articles also reside in *Health Research Policy and Systems,* 2009, 7(Suppl. 1), published December 16, 2009. Here are the series articles and authors:

- "SUPPORT Tools for Evidence-Informed Health Policymaking (STP)," by John N. Lavis, Andrew D. Oxman, Simon Lewin, and Atle Fretheim

- "SUPPORT Tools for Evidence-Informed Health Policymaking (STP) 1: What Is Evidence-Informed Policymaking?" by Andrew D. Oxman, John N. Lavis, Simon Lewin, and Atle Fretheim

- "SUPPORT Tools for Evidence-Informed Health Policymaking (STP) 2: Improving How Your Organization Supports the Use of Research Evidence to Inform Policymaking," by Andrew D. Oxman, Per Olav Vandvik, John N. Lavis, Atle Fretheim, and Simon Lewin

- "SUPPORT Tools for Evidence-Informed Health Policymaking (STP) 3: Setting Priorities for Supporting Evidence-Informed Policymaking," by John N. Lavis, Andrew D. Oxman, Simon Lewin, and Atle Fretheim

- "SUPPORT Tools for Evidence-Informed Health Policymaking (STP) 4: Using Research Evidence to Clarify a Problem," by John N. Lavis, Michael G. Wilson, Andrew D. Oxman, Simon Lewin, and Atle Fretheim

- "SUPPORT Tools for Evidence-Informed Health Policymaking (STP) 5: Using Research Evidence to Frame Options to Address a Problem," by John N. Lavis, Michael G. Wilson, Andrew D. Oxman, Jeremy Grimshaw, Simon Lewin, and Atle Fretheim

- "SUPPORT Tools for Evidence-Informed Health Policymaking (STP) 6: Using Research Evidence to Address How an Option Will Be Implemented," by Atle Fretheim, Susan Munabi-Babigumira, Andrew D. Oxman, John N. Lavis, and Simon Lewin

- "SUPPORT Tools for Evidence-Informed Health Policymaking (STP) 7: Finding Systematic Reviews," by John N. Lavis, Andrew D. Oxman, Jeremy Grimshaw, Marit Johansen, Jennifer A. Boyko, Simon Lewin, and Atle Fretheim

- "SUPPORT Tools for Evidence-Informed Health Policymaking (STP) 8: Deciding How Much Confidence to Place in a Systematic Review," by Simon Lewin, Andrew D. Oxman, John N. Lavis, and Atle Fretheim

- "SUPPORT Tools for Evidence-Informed Health Policymaking (STP) 9: Assessing the Applicability of the Findings of a Systematic Review," by John N. Lavis, Andrew D. Oxman, Nathan M. Souza, Simon Lewin, Russell L. Gruen, and Atle Fretheim

- "SUPPORT Tools for Evidence-Informed Health Policymaking (STP) 10: Taking Equity Into Consideration When Assessing the Findings of a Systematic Review," by Andrew D. Oxman, John N. Lavis, Simon Lewin, and Atle Fretheim

- "SUPPORT Tools for Evidence-Informed Health Policymaking (STP) 11: Finding and Using Evidence About Local Conditions," by Simon Lewin, Andrew D. Oxman, John N. Lavis, Atle Fretheim, Sebastian Garcia Marti, and Susan Munabi-Babigumira

- "SUPPORT Tools for Evidence-Informed Health Policymaking (STP) 12: Finding and Using Research Evidence About Resource Use and Costs," by Andrew D. Oxman, Atle Fretheim, John N. Lavis, and Simon Lewin

- "SUPPORT Tools for Evidence-Informed Health Policymaking (STP) 13: Preparing and Using Policy Briefs to Support Evidence-Informed Policymaking," by John N. Lavis, Govin Permanand, Andrew D. Oxman, Simon Lewin, and Atle Fretheim

- "SUPPORT Tools for Evidence-Informed Health Policymaking (STP) 14: Organising and Using Policy Dialogues to Support Evidence-Informed Policymaking," by John N. Lavis, Jennifer A. Boyko, Andrew D. Oxman, Simon Lewin, and Atle Fretheim

- "SUPPORT Tools for Evidence-Informed Health Policymaking (STP) 15: Engaging the Public in Evidence-Informed Policymaking," by Andrew D. Oxman, Simon Lewin, John N. Lavis, and Atle Fretheim

- "SUPPORT Tools for Evidence-Informed Health Policymaking (STP) 16: Using Research Evidence in Balancing the Pros and Cons of Policies," by Andrew D. Oxman, John N. Lavis, Atle Fretheim, and Simon Lewin

- "SUPPORT Tools for Evidence-Informed Health Policymaking (STP) 17: Dealing With Insufficient Research Evidence," by Andrew D. Oxman, John N. Lavis, Atle Fretheim, and Simon Lewin

- "SUPPORT Tools for Evidence-Informed Health Policymaking (STP) 18: Planning Monitoring and Evaluation of Policies," by Atle Fretheim, Andrew D. Oxman, John N. Lavis, and Simon Lewin

References

AcademyHealth. (2018). Moving evidence into action. Retrieved from https://www.academy-health.org/

Alexander, P. E., Gionfriddo, M. R., Li, S. A., Bero, L., Stoltzfus, R. J., Neuman, I., . . . Guyatt, G. H. (2016). A number of factors explain why WHO guideline developers make strong recommendations inconsistent with GRADE guidance. *Journal of Clinical Epidemiology, 70*, 111–122. doi:10.1016/j.jclinepi.2015.09.006

GRADE. (n.d.). Welcome to the GRADE working group. Retrieved from http://www.gradeworkinggroup.org/

Guyatt, G., Oxman, A. D., Akl, E. A., Kunz, R., Vist, G., Brozek, J., . . . Schünemann, H. J. (2011). GRADE guidelines: 1. introduction-GRADE evidence profiles and summary of findings tables. *Journal of Clinical Epidemiology, 64*(4), 383–394. doi:10.1016/j.jclinepi.2010.04.026

Guyatt, G. H., Oxman, A. D., Vist, G. E., Kunz, R., Falck-Ytter, Y., Alonso-Coello, P., …GRADE working group. (2008). GRADE: An emerging consensus on rating quality of evidence and strength of recommendations. *British Medical Journal, 336*, 924–926. doi:10.1136/bmj.39489.470347.AD

Oxman, A. D., & Hanney, S. (2009). SUPPORT tools for evidence-informed health policymaking (STP). *Health Research Policy and Systems, 7*(Suppl. 1), S1.

Oxman, A. D., Lavis, J. N., & Fretheim, A. (2007). Use of evidence in WHO recommendations. *The Lancet, 369*(9576), 1883–1889. doi:10.1016/S0140-6736(07)60675-8

Schünemann, H. J., Fretheim, A., Oxman, A. D., & WHO Advisory Committee on Health Research. (2006). Improving the use of research evidence in guideline development: 1. guidelines for guidelines. *Health Research Policy and Systems, 4*(13).

B

GLOBAL EXAMPLES OF EVIDENCE-INFORMED POLICYMAKING: AN ANNOTATED BIBLIOGRAPHY

This appendix provides a non-exhaustive annotated bibliography of evidence-informed policymaking and processes from around the globe. Because the focus of this book is on policymaking in the United States, these examples have been selected from regions around the world. However, this bibliography ends with several multi-region collaborative papers; two of these include resources from the US.

This annotated bibliography is organized alphabetically by continent/world region. Each example begins with its title and date of publication. Following you will find the names of authors, publication information, and access information. Open access article links are provided where available.

Africa

Ghana

Informing Evidence-Based Policies for Ageing and Health in Ghana (2015)

Authors	Islene Araujo de Carvalho, Julie Byles, Charles Aquah, George Amofah, Richard Biritwum, Ulysses Panisset, James Goodwin, and John Beard
Publication	*Bulletin of the World Health Organization, 93*(1), 47–51
DOI	10.2471/BLT.14.136242
Open Access URL	https://www.ncbi.nlm.nih.gov/pmc/articles/PMC4271679/

This article describes the evidence-based policymaking approach used in Ghana, with technical support from the World Health Organization (WHO), to address priority health problems related to Ghana's aging population. The WHO's knowledge translation framework on ageing and health was used to underpin a four-step process, which involved the following:

1. Defining priority problems and health-system responses via a country assessment using epidemiologic data, policy review, site visits, and key informant interviews

2. Gathering evidence on effective health systems interventions in low-, middle-, and high-income countries

3. Conducting a policy dialogue in which key stakeholders were engaged

4. Developing policy briefs, which were presented to the Ghana Health Service in 2014

The authors identify six priority problem areas. Of these, stakeholders agreed with five; policy options were then developed around those five areas. In the article, the authors address facilitators and challenges to the process and conclude by discussing how the WHO's knowledge translation framework for ageing and health could be of use in these settings and for this purpose.

Malawi

Malaria Research and Its Influence on Anti-Malarial Drug Policy in Malawi: A Case Study (2016)

Authors	Chikondi Mwendera, Christiaan de Jager, Herbert Longwe, Kamija Phiri, Charles Hongoro, and Clifford M. Mutero
Publication	*Health Research Policy and Systems, 14,* 41
DOI	10.1186/s12961-016-0108-1
Open Access URL	https://www.ncbi.nlm.nih.gov/pubmed/27246503

This article chronicles the process used to retrospectively examine the appropriateness of a policy change in the guidelines for treating malaria in sub-Saharan Africa, using a body of evidence and key informant insights. The Malawi first-line treatment for uncomplicated malaria changed in 1993 from chloroquine to sulfadoxine-pyrimethamine (SP), and from SP to lumefantrine-artemether in 2007. The authors undertook this evidence-based health policy case study because concerns had been raised about the 1993 change and whether it had led to the development of Plasmodium falciparum resistance to SP. The authors used a systematic review to examine the evidence between 1984 and 1993, when chloroquine was the first-line drug of choice, and between 1994 and 2007, when the first-line drug of choice was SP. Key informant interviews accompany the systematic reviews; participants were asked specific questions about the policy change with regard to availability and adequacy of evidence for decision-making at the time, the timing of the policy changes, the justifiability of the change, and any challenges encountered. The article concludes that ample evidence justified the policy changes and affirms the necessity of locally generated evidence when making such a policy change.

Nigeria

The Challenge of Bridging the Gap Between Researchers and Policy Makers: Experiences of a Health Policy Research Group in Engaging Policy Makers to Support Evidence Informed Policy Making in Nigeria (2016)

Authors	Benjamin Uzochukwu, Obinna Onwujekwe, Chinyere Mbachu, Chinenye Okwuosa, Enyi Etiaba, Monica E. Nyström, and Lucy Gilson
Publication	*Globalization and Health, 12*, 67
DOI	10.1186/s12992-016-0209-1
Open Access URL	https://globalizationandhealth.biomedcentral.com/articles/10.1186/s12992-016-0209-1

This paper is an analysis of experiences culled from seven cases in which studies by the Health Policy Research Group sought to influence policy approaches in three states of Nigeria. In-depth interviews with policymakers and researchers were used to explore the experiences. Results are represented in a model using the getting research into policy and practice (GRIPP) process, and challenges to research utilization in health policy are reported. Among these are the policymakers' demands for research, their uptake of research, and the communication gap that exists between researchers, donors, and policymakers. Additional challenges reported include the political process itself, that some policymakers were unwilling to use research, that funding for research was limited, and resistance to change.

Uganda

Malaria Treatment Policy Change in Uganda: What Role Did Evidence Play? (2014)

Authors	Juliet Nabyonga-Orem, Freddie Ssengooba, Jean Macq, and Bart Criel
Publication	*Malaria Journal, 13*, 345
DOI	10.1186/1475-2875-13-345
Open Access URL	https://malariajournal.biomedcentral.com/articles/10.1186/1475-2875-13-345

This paper is a follow-up to earlier work on malaria in Uganda. It uses a case-study approach as well as mixed methods to understand the complex contextual issues surrounding a change in the malaria treatment policy that occurred over a 25-month period between March 2004 and April 2006. The aim of the study was to identify the nature of evidence uptake related to the malaria policy change. The most important facilitating factors in the uptake of evidence were found to be availability of high quality/contextualized evidence, including its effective dissemination; Ministry of Health leadership in the process, with mutual trust and availability of funding tools; and inputs to implement evidence. Barriers included resistance from implementers, the capacity of the health system to implement evidence, and financial sustainability.

Middle East/Western Asia

Iran

Development of Evidence-Based Health Policy Documents in Developing Countries: A Case of Iran (2014)

Authors	Mohammad Hasan Imani-Nasab, Hesam Seyedin, Reza Majdzadeh, Bahareh Yazdizadeh, and Masoud Salehi
Publication	*Global Journal of Health Science*, 6(3), 27–36
DOI	10.5539/gjhs.v6n3p27
Open Access URL	https://www.ncbi.nlm.nih.gov/pmc/articles/PMC4825355/

The aim of this qualitative study was to examine perspectives about barriers and facilitators in developing evidence-based health policy documents (EBPDs) in a developing country, from the point of view of the producers of the EBPDs. The study was theory-based, using the theory of planned behavior. Methods employed included semi-structured interviews. The sample was selected using purposive and snowball sampling. The researchers found that, despite concerns about time consumption and contextualization, participants held positive attitudes toward the development of EBPDs. Not all stakeholders supported EBPDs, however. Main barriers to EBPD development were related to control beliefs, which, according to the theory base, are those related to organization and health systems levels.

Palestine

Understanding the Concept and Importance of the Health Research System in Palestine: A Qualitative Study (2018)

Authors	Mohammed AlKhaldi, Yehia Abed, Constanze Pfeiffer, Saleem Haj-Yahia, Abdulsalam Alkaiyat, and Marcel Tanner
Publication	*Health Research Policy and Systems, 16*(1), 49
DOI	10.1186/s12961-018-0315-z
Open Access URL	https://www.ncbi.nlm.nih.gov/pubmed/29914533

This study assessed the perceptions of policymakers, academics, and experts of the concept of health research systems (HRS). This is an emerging concept in Palestine and helps address health-related challenges. Three sectors were studied using in-depth interviews and focus groups: policymakers, academics, and directors and experts. Findings demonstrated that most participants agreed that HRS was a positive factor associated with improvement and that its neglect was perceived as a loss. Data analysis also revealed that health experts in Palestine had an inadequate understanding of HRS, which is a barrier to application. In addition, findings demonstrated support for a central governing body to promote awareness and for strengthening the understanding of HRS in Palestine.

Assessing Policy-Makers,' Academics' and Experts' Satisfaction With the Performance of the Palestinian Health Research System: A Qualitative Study (2018)

Authors	Mohammed AlKhaldi, Yehia Abed, Constanze Pfeiffer, Saleem Haj-Yahia, Abdulsalam Alkaiyat, and Marcel Tanner
Publication	*Health Research Policy and Systems, 16*(1), 66
DOI	10.1186/s12961-018-0341-x
Open Access URL	https://health-policy-systems.biomedcentral.com/articles/10.1186/s12961-018-0341-x

This paper, by the same authors as the previous paper, describes a study carried out in three sectors in Palestine, different from those in the first paper. The researchers examined the satisfaction of policymakers, academics, and experts with the overall performance of health research systems (HRS). It also investigated their perceptions regarding political will and attention to the utilization of health research. The aim of the study was to identify gaps related to performance and to produce insights on how to strengthen HRS performance. The three sectors in which the study was carried out were government institutions, public health universities, and major local and international health nongovernmental organizations. Semi-structured in-depth interviews and focus-group discussions were conducted; thematic analysis was used to describe findings. The researchers concluded that the Palestinian HRS is underperforming, as perceived by the health experts interviewed, and that research is not on the government leadership's agenda. Recommendations to engage health decision-makers and establish a strategic plan are put forward based on the findings.

Western Europe

Scotland

Implementing Health Policy: Lessons From the Scottish Well Men's Policy Initiative (2015)

Authors	Flora Douglas, Edwin van Teijlingen, Cairns Smith, and Mandy Moffat
Publication	*AIMS Public Health, 2*(4), 887–905
DOI	10.3934/publichealth.2015.4.887
Open Access URL	http://aura.abdn.ac.uk/handle/2164/5325

This article reports on a qualitative evaluation of the implementation of the Well Men's Services (WMS) policy initiative by the Scottish government to address men's health inequalities. Scottish men have a lower average life expectancy than men in other parts of the United Kingdom, and mortality rates are poor in Scotland even when compared to parts of Eastern Europe. The most cited explanations for men's health inequalities are associated with lifestyle behaviors and that men use health services sub-optimally compared to women, make less use of primary healthcare services, and delay seeking healthcare. In response, the WMS policy initiative was funded with a focus on making health and social care services more effective, particularly for hard-to-reach and disadvantaged men. Seven multi-agency health, social care, and volunteer agencies located in urban, rural, and remote island areas were selected for project funding. These coalitions developed and delivered 16 separate projects focused on the target population. This analysis was conducted to investigate the realities of policy implementation in the real-world setting compared with principles of rational planning tenets. The post-hoc mixed-method qualitative analysis used a sample of national policymakers; local health and social care professionals were interviewed regarding their perceptions. Findings revealed four key themes:

- There was ambiguity about the policy problem and how the intervention was to proceed.

- Behavioral framing of the policy problem and intervention was important.

- There was uncertainty regarding the evidence base upon which the policy was created and its outcomes.

- There was a focus on the intervention as the outcome.

In their conclusion, the authors suggest the following:

- A new approach to planning and implementing these types of public health interventions must recognize the complexity and political nature of the health problems the policy seeks to ameliorate.

- Evidence regarding intervention will be imperfect and contested.

- New approaches must consider future associated uncertainties.

Sweden

Recentralizing Healthcare Through Evidence-Based Guidelines–Striving for National Equity in Sweden (2014)

Authors	Mio Fredriksson, Paula Blomqvist, and Ulrika Winblad
Publication	*BMC Health Services Research, 14,* 509
DOI	10.1186/s12913-014-0509-1
Open Access URL	https://bmchealthservres.biomedcentral.com/articles/10.1186/s12913-014-0509-1

This paper describes an evaluation of the evidence-based Swedish National (health) Guidelines. Along with Sweden's national medical registries and a system of quality and efficiency indicators, these guidelines form Sweden's quality-management system. These guidelines were evaluated using a framework for evaluation and comparison-making. The researchers concluded that Sweden's evidence-based guidelines should be seen in the context of Sweden's constitutional setting, which involves several levels of autonomous political authority. As healthcare is being recentralized in Sweden and the scope for local decision-making reduced, this evaluation is an important part of the process.

United Kingdom

Are UK Governments Utilizing the Most Effective Evidence-Based Policies for Ill-Health Prevention? (2017)

Authors	British Medical Association
Publication	British Medical Association
DOI	N/A
Open Access URL	https://www.bma.org.uk/-/media/files/pdfs/ collective%20voice/policy%20research/public %20and%20population%20health/are-uk-governments -using-evidence-based-policies-ill-health-prevention.pdf

This paper is both a critique and a review of the literature and findings of the state of evidence-based policies for ill-health prevention in the UK. The UK government, through its National Health Service (NHS), has been the provider of health services for some time. Poor public health across the UK has contributed to an increased demand for healthcare services, which has led to increasing financial and operational pressures on the NHS. While this has resulted in commitments to focus on preventive healthcare, this document purports that a priority to engage an evidence-based approach has not been actualized and that the use of evidence in public health policy has been inconsistent. The British Medical Association suggests there is justification for government regulation to support population health improvements. Several population health measures and their strengths and weaknesses are reported. Among these are actions to reduce smoking rates, regulate alcohol, regulate sugar reduction as it relates to childhood obesity, and establish standard packaging for tobacco products. This paper concludes that reasons for the inconsistent use of evidence are multifactorial. These include an absence of political will and differences in the changing and devolving powers across the UK. Competing interests of commercial companies are also factors worth considering.

South Asia

India

Voices of Decision Makers on Evidence-Based Policy: A Case of Evolving TB/HIV Co-Infection Policy in India (2016)

Authors	K. Srikanth Reddy and Seema Sahay
Publication	*AIDS Care, 28*(3), 397–400
DOI	10.1080/09540121.2015.1096889
Open Access URL	N/A

This study explored the perspectives of policy decision-makers on the use of evidence in TB/HIV policymaking in India. The TB co-infection incidence in HIV-infected individuals is rising, and policy for prevention and treatment for those individuals is evolving. This study used purposive sampling to interview key national and international policy decision-makers in India about this policymaking process. Findings showed that although decision-makers relied on global evidence because it was readily available, local evidence was essential. This was because global evidence was not necessarily the best information to apply in-context and therefore was not the best evidence upon which to base local policy decisions. Multi-center studies in the country in which the policy would be instituted were found to be all-important. Findings also showed a gap in the interface between researchers and policymakers, that researchers should design research that is relevant to policymaking, and that communication between researchers and policymakers should be more flexible and consultative.

Oceana

Australia

Web-Based Geo-Visualisation of Spatial Information to Support Evidence-Based Health Policy: A Case Study of the Development Process of *HealthTracks* (2014)

Authors	Andrew Jardine, Narelle Mullan, Ori Gudes, James Cosford, Simon Moncrieff, Geoff West, Jianguo Xiao, Grace Yun, and Peter Somerford
Publication	*Health Information Management Journal, 43*(2), 7–16
DOI	10.1177/183335831404300202
Open Access URL	N/A

This article describes the *HealthTracks* project, which brings multiple data sources together in an online geo-visualization. Its use is to gather spatial health information, necessary for revealing disease spread and clustering of patterns associated with risk factors and areas of need. This information is then available to health policy decision-makers, such as policymakers, analysts, planners, and program managers across the Department of Health Western Australia. The authors discuss future expansion plans for *HealthTracks*, including increasing the range of data available and the development of new analytical capabilities.

Multi-Region/Collaborative Papers

Africa With Germany and Other Partners

An Approach for Setting Evidence-Based and Stakeholder-Informed Research Priorities in Low- and Middle-Income Countries (2016)

Authors	Eva A. Rehfuess, Solange Durão, Patrick Kyamanywa, Joerg J. Meerpohl, Taryn Young, and Anke Rohwer on behalf of the CEBHA+ and consortium
Publication	*Bulletin of the World Health Organization, 94*, 297–305
DOI	10.2471/BLT.15.162966
Open Access URL	https://www.ncbi.nlm.nih.gov/pmc/articles/ PMC4794302/pdf/BLT.15.162966.pdf

This paper describes the pragmatic approach used to set evidence-based and stakeholder-informed research priorities in Africa by the Collaboration for Evidence-Based Healthcare and Public Health in Africa (CEBHA+). The CEBHA+ is a consortium of eight partners in five countries (Ethiopia, Malawi, Rwanda, South Africa, and Uganda), two German partners, and two associate partners. The purposes for establishing a pragmatic approach were to ensure that research to inform policymaking would achieve the following:

- Avoid duplication and fill research gaps in the existing African/international evidence base
- Be relevant to address questions asked by decision-makers
- Be context-sensitive to usability in African settings
- Be feasible with regard to utilization
- Be of high quality

A stepped approach was used to develop research priorities, further identify top priorities from the priority list, develop priority research questions, and develop concomitant evidence maps. Two evidence maps on diabetes and hypertension and one on road traffic injuries were developed; another on tuberculosis-HIV was begun but not completed. Study protocols were developed to address each priority research question. This pragmatic process was found to be useful, strengthened research collaboration within and across continents, and facilitated the expansion of long-term capacity and infrastructure for health and public health policy based on evidence in sub-Saharan Africa.

Australia, the UK, and the USA

Using Population-Based Routine Data for Evidence-Based Health Policy Decisions: Lessons From Three Examples of Setting and Evaluating National Health Policy in Australia, the UK and the USA (2007)

Authors	Elaine H. Morrato, Melinda Elias, and Christian A. Gericke
Publication	*Journal of Public Health*, *29*(4), 463–471
DOI	10.1093/pubmed/fdm065
Open Access URL	N/A

This paper describes three case studies in which population-based data were used to inform national health policy in three different countries. The cases relate to prescription drug safety (USA), childhood immunization (Australia), and hospital waiting times (UK). The goal of the paper was to summarize general lessons learned about using population-based databases to inform policymaking. Important lessons across the cases included the importance of political will in initiating data collection, sustaining data-collection efforts, and conducting analysis at a national level. Additionally, the paper addresses the kinds of decision-making factors databases can address, as well as how data was integrated into the decision-making process. The authors conclude that population-based databases can provide important information for policy decision-makers. Important database uses include identifying populations that are most vulnerable and using the information to develop policy goals and to track and evaluate health policy intervention effectiveness.

The Netherlands (With Experience in East Africa)

Using Knowledge Brokering to Promote Evidence-Based Policy-Making: The Need for Support Structures (2006)

Authors	Jessica van Kammen, Don de Savigny, and Nelson Sewankambo
Publication	*Bulletin of the World Health Organization, 84*(8), 608–612
DOI	N/A
Open Access URL	https://www.scielosp.org/article/bwho/2006.v84n8/608-612/

The authors describe the usefulness of knowledge brokering as an approach and strategy to bridge the know-do gap in health policymaking. Knowledge brokering addresses the issues inherent in evidence-based policymaking: that researchers produce scientific evidence that might not be tailored to the context of the policy in question, that the evidence is characterized by complexity and uncertainty, and that policymakers may not be able to convey their specific contexts or policy challenges to allow for the time to produce research to answer their questions. This paper describes two experiences in which knowledge brokering was successfully used. One example was to inform a policy on subfertility care in the Netherlands; the other was the experience of the Regional East African Community Health Policy Initiative. The authors identify the characteristics of knowledge brokering, describe the stepped processes in each example, and conclude that support structures are essential for success in the process.

The United States and Canada

A Call for Evidence-Based Medical Treatment of Opioid Dependence in the United States and Canada (2013)

Authors	Bohdan Nosyk, M. Douglas Anglin, Suzanne Brissette, Thomas Kerr, David C. Marsh, Bruce R. Schackman, Evan Wood, and Julio S. G. Montaner
Publication	*Health Affairs, 32*(8), 1462–1469
DOI	10.1377/hlthaff.2012.0846
Open Access URL	https://www.healthaffairs.org/doi/10.1377/hlthaff.2012.0846#

This paper is not an example but an analysis and commentary on the underuse of medical treatment for opioid dependence in North America and a subsequent call for appropriate evidence-based, policy-driven medical treatment. The authors, representing institutions in the US and Canada, provide a review of the literature and persuasive arguments for the two countries to conform to best practice suggested by the existing body of evidence. They identify that the largest cause for the gap between practice and evidence-based standards in both countries is related to both regulatory restraints and pervasive sub-optimal clinical practices. Based on the body of evidence, one of the recommendations made by the authors is the elimination of the restrictions on office-based methadone prescribing in the US. In addition, evidence-based policy actions such as reducing financial barriers to treatment, reducing reliance on less effective treatment and potentially unsafe treatment (such as opioid detoxification), and exploring the integration of emerging treatments are recommended.

INDEX

A

B

G

H

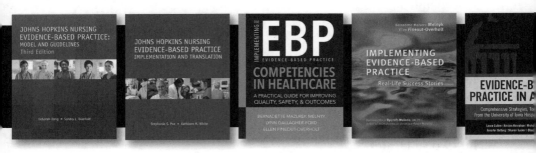
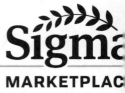

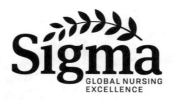

Sigma brings home more awards!

CHECK OUT OUR 2018 *AMERICAN JOURNAL OF NURSING (AJN)* BOOK OF THE YEAR AWARDS

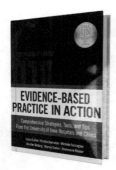

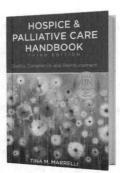

Evidence-Based Practice in Action
(9781940446936)

Second Place

**Education/Continuing Education/
Professional Development category**

Hospice & Palliative Care Handbook,
Third Edition
(9781945157455)

Second Place

Palliative Care and Hospice category

See Sigma's 2017 *AJN* Book of the Year Award recipients

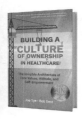

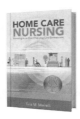

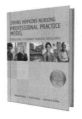

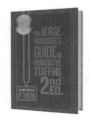

Building a Culture
of Ownership in
Healthcare

First Place

Home Care
Nursing

Second Place

Johns Hopkins Nursing
Professional Practice
Model

Second Place

The Nurse Manager's
Guide to Innovative
Staffing, Second Edition

Third Place

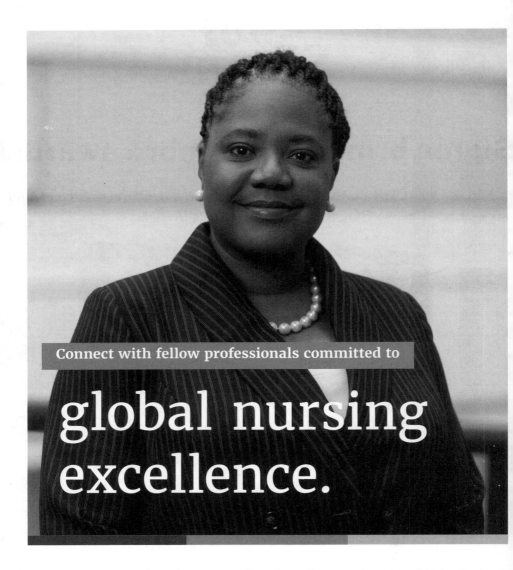

Connect with fellow professionals committed to

global nursing excellence.

At Sigma, we develop nurse leaders like you by providing the resources and opportunities to support you throughout your nursing career.

Together, our dedicated members change lives and advance healthcare.

Learn how you can be a Sigma member at
https://Join.SigmaNursing.org.

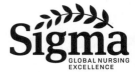